EFFICIENCY-IMPROVING INNOVATIONS IN SOCIAL CARE OF THE ELDERLY

Efficiency-Improving Innovations in Social Care of the Elderly

EWAN FERLIE
DAVID CHALLIS
BLEDDYN DAVIES

Gower

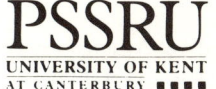

Published by
Avebury
Gower Publishing Company Limited
Gower House
Croft Road
Aldershot
Hants GU11 3HR
England

Gower Publishing Company
Old Post Road
Brookfield
Vermont 05036
USA

British Library Cataloguing in Publication Data

Ferlie, Ewan, *1956–*
    Efficiency improving innovations in community
    care of the elderly.
    1. Great Britain. Old persons. Community care
    I. Title   II. Challis, David, *1948–*   III.
    Davies, Bleddyn, *1936–*
    362.6′1′0941

ISBN 0–566–07049–9

Printed by Athenæum Press
Newcastle upon Tyne

Contents

viii

Tables

Preface

This book is one of the products of an interest in efficiency-improving innovations in the community-based care of the elderly first developed at the PSSRU almost a decade ago. The DHSS asked the Unit to undertake a sweep of innovations in social services departments. From this, Ewan Ferlie, then a new research associate, made and edited a compendium of descriptions written by agency personnel closely connected with the innovation. This *Directory of Initiatives* (Ferlie, 1980) was published by the PSSRU.

It was clear that the *Directory* material would be an invaluable basis for analysing the nature of social service innovation; of course, as with the traveller asking the way to Dublin, a less than ideal place from which to start, but the spot where our DHSS obligations had located us. The analysis of their characteristics would be particularly valuable at a time when fiscal, political and policy environments were changing fast: expenditure cuts, a new government promising fundamental changes in the roles of the State at central and local levels, a new managerialist argument emerging from academics and the highest levels of government with greater stress on efficiency and successful implementation. Social services departments were both reacting against some of the *hubris* which accompanied the immediate post-Seebohm growth in resources and accretion of responsibilities and working through the communitarian assumptions of the Seebohm era. So we analysed the *Directory* data (i) to tease out elements which the innovators expected would cause their innovative arrangements to

1

have beneficial outcomes — to describe how innovators thought their schemes would improve equity and efficiency; (ii) to analyse the process of innovation; (iii) to investigate how contextual variation affected the frequency and nature of innovations; (iv) to develop a typology of innovations, and (v) to investigate whether policy devices increased the frequency and affected the nature of innovations. The first analyses showed that the method yielded interesting argument. Therefore the authors made a second collection of information about innovations. The collection was extended to cover agencies other than social services departments. On this was based the *Sourcebook of Innovations in the Community Care of the Elderly* (Ferlie, 1982) and *A Guide to Efficiency-Improving Innovations in the Care of the Frail Elderly* (Ferlie, Challis and Davies, 1983), a Michelin *Guide* to the community-based social care with the logic of each scheme summarised by a classification of characteristics but presented in a modern format. The argument was later incorporated into the Unit's programme on continuity and change in community-based service, the most recent publications being chapters in *Resources, Needs and Outcomes in Community-Based Care* (Bebbington, Davies and associates, 1989). Ewan Ferlie gave almost all his time to the study of efficiency-improving innovations for some years. He is the principal author of this book.

The Study as Bureaumetric Analysis of Equity and Efficiency

The development of quantitative indicators to analyse organisational characteristics has in recent years been given a glossy name: 'bureaumetrics' (Hood and Dunsire, 1981). The classification of characteristics is key to the published papers and also to this book, and we would have thought it wasteful not to have undertaken statistical analysis. The nature of the evidence, accounts of many ventures, a wide collection of evidence produced by correspondents from the schemes but edited by us after telephone discussion and correspondence, focused our attention on anatomy and rationale rather than physiology and process. The data pushed us towards the bureaumetric analysis of structure rather than the anthropological observation of the evolution of structure, process and assumptive worlds in their bargaining, power and learning contexts. Our analysis developed an extension of the Aston school's style of contingency analysis, studying the interrelationship of indicators of a set of structural features of organisations and their influence on outcomes. Therefore, we found ourselves to be more like Molière's M. Jourdain than the character himself: not only speaking bureaumetrics for many years without realising it, but bureaumetrics which by the standards of administrative studies had quite an elaborate theoretical framework, posing questions whose answers required the application of statistical modelling.

Inevitably, the framework reflected the PSSRU's production relations approach: the focus was equity and efficiency, and process questions were asked only to illuminate argument about why the equity and efficiency outcomes could be improved. Primarily, we were seeking links between the arrangements in innovatory schemes and improvements in the equity and efficiency of outcomes. Only secondarily did we wish to illuminate the organisational processes associated with the process of innovation and its subsequent translation into standard arrangements. We argued that the link between arrangements and equity and efficiency outcomes could be achieved either by the better matching of existing resources to needs, in effect the performance of the core tasks of case management, or by changing the resources, in effect changing the inputs of the services themselves. This distinction reflected the PSSRU's experimental investigations of the effects of entrepreneurial case management (Challis and Davies, 1986; Davies and Challis, 1986) and its development from the original American argument of a normative theory of case management; a strand of argument more recently reflected in the Care in the Community initiative, the Griffiths and Wagner reports, the writings of the Audit Commission and the Social Services Inspectorate (DHSS, 1983; Griffiths, 1988; Wagner, 1988; Audit Commission, 1987; Social Services Inspectorate, 1987).

Publications from the Study not Subsequently Mentioned

This book is the latest of a series of publications. It might be useful to be reminded of their foci, since their argument is not repeated elsewhere in the book.

- Davies (1981b) drew on the findings to argue that innovations are mostly geographically very localised, seldom specific with respect to target clientele, and disjointed rather than related moves in co-ordinated system-wide change. The paper argued for greater clarity in defining the core functions of government and departmental effort to improve cost-effectiveness of outcomes, and the provision of the preconditions for individuals to discharge essential responsibilities increasingly resourcefully and so the preconditions to encourage innovation.
- Davies and Ferlie (1982) used the classification to describe the

3

nature of innovations, and the probabilities that types of innovation would survive stages of the process from conception to
having widespread and permanent effect on agency activity. It
showed how the frequency of innovation reflected the characteristics and circumstances of authorities. Among its findings were
that authorities conducting service reviews tended to raise
resources for innovation from outside agencies, particularly joint
finance from the health authorities; that the frequency was higher
in larger authorities; and that authorities with high expenditures
and continuing growth were less likely to make innovations
financed from their own funds. The pattern of innovations during
the period were almost panic reactions to the spending crises of
the later 1970s. A similar analysis of data from the second sweep
suggested that the nature of innovations had changed. Some of
the innovations which were at the leading edge three years earlier
were by then the most common types. Fewer were the immediate
responses to cuts. Indeed, the development of the community
services as the basis for a more efficient pattern of social care had
become a major feature of innovatory activity, and reflected long-
term trends in arguments about system development rather than
the panic reaction to a financial crisis. Growing resources encouraged internally financed innovation.

- Ferlie, Challis and Davies (1984) described ideal-typical forms of
innovation found in the second sweep, estimated the frequency
of each type, and showed how they reflected their institutional
sponsorship, and so sponsors' interests, other features of their
assumptive worlds, and the structural features creating incentives,
opportunities and constraints. The paper illustrated the importance of the few schemes whose arguments and arrangement were
exciting enough to have an important influence on future development. For instance, there were a few which made the improvement
in the performance of more than one or two of the core tasks of
case management central to their logics. (Schemes embodying the
improvement of assessment were more common — as would be
hoped, since multidisciplinary assessment was by then as near to
being DHSS practice policy as one finds in social care.) The
analysis distinguished one type which was of great interest in the
light of subsequent argument about the development of
community care because it required interprofessional co-operation
often led by geriatricians but making social workers in effect case
managers of more intensive and flexible services.

- Ferlie, Challis and Davies (1985) focused on the differences in the
second sweep between schemes financed from the base budget
and joint finance. The results were less gloomy than might be

inferred from some contemporary comments about the programme. The process evidence we had collected suggested that they were likely to achieve efficiency gains, although it seemed likely that schemes would vary in the extent of their achievement. We saw less of the backlash against joint finance than was then argued. Indeed, we argued for what was in effect the development from the joint consultative committees (JCCs) and joint finance mechanisms: a budget-holding agency for clients requiring both long-term medical and social care inputs linking health and social care personnel, a concept later suggested by the Audit Commission (1986).

- Most recently, a chapter in *Resources, Needs and Outcomes in Community-Based Care* (Bebbington, Davies and associates, 1989) was based on the closer study of innovations in a dozen social services departments in England and Wales. Data about resource utilisation, needs-related circumstances and outcomes were collected mainly by interviewing 500 cases and their principal carers. Evidence about structures, policies and assumptive worlds and their recent history was collated from agency documents and by interviewing officers and field workers. So the analysis was of fewer schemes in greater depth. Its primary purpose continued to be to contribute to the development of the production of welfare approach, but its data collection allowed a more illuminating analysis of structure and process than had previously been possible.

Individual Schemes and their Characteristics

We found that putting the evidence and argument between one pair of covers produced a manuscript which was long and mixed the interests of quite different target readerships. Therefore this book includes only the essentials of the argument. We have printed a second volume, consisting mainly of detailed analyses of each of the innovatory schemes. This we believe to be the most comprehensive analytic listing and description of schemes available, and we expect it to be useful to both the policy and academic worlds. *Efficiency-Improving Innovations in the Community Care of Frail Elderly People: Individual Schemes and their Characteristics* is available from the Executive Officer, PSSRU, University of Kent at Canterbury, England CT2 7NF.

Current and Future Work

The signs and symptoms approach to diagnosis can often mislead; more often in the analysis of the consequences of change for the equity and efficiency of outcomes in social care than in most branches of medicine, we hope. However, it is in both contexts much cheaper than more reliable alternatives. It would be useful to test our indicators for the degree of correlation between process and outcome. Our more recent work has analysed resources, the needs-related circumstances of clients and carers and outcomes for them of innovatory schemes and more standard provision as well as study the nature of innovations and their inception and development, as can be seen from *Resources, Needs and Outcomes* (Bebbington, Davies and associates, 1989). Future work will follow the same strategy — though this is not easy, since econometric analysis and other methods of studying personal social service organisations mix oil with water at every stage from designing a study to stating the argument developed from its results. Increasingly the focus is on the management of change and is based on very general investigations of many agencies supported by the in-depth study of a few.

Innovations must not be viewed apart from the wider environmental and organisational continuities and changes. The key issues are well known: how management can influence organisational cultures and more specifically the willingness to embrace change, and how it can create the opportunities and incentives to make changes which improve the equity and efficiency of outcomes of a system which is complex in the multeity and variety of its organisational divisions, agencies, organisational levels, occupational interests and perspectives. The study of innovations *per se* is important in the wider research agenda both for what it tells us about the broader issues and because it is through innovations that some of the broadest systemic objectives will be achieved; for example, in schemes for decanting persons from long-stay hospitals described in *Care in the Community: the First Steps* (Renshaw, Hampson, Thomason, Darton, Judge and Knapp, 1988) and *Demonstrating Successful Care in the Community* (Knapp and Cambridge, 1988). Implementation questions seem to many in the policy world to be the most important of all in this new managerialist age.

Acknowledgements

Our liaison officers, initially Jack Barnes, then Hazel Canter, and during the final preparation for publication, Sue Moylan, have as always helped in innumerable ways which are invisible to those whose research is not commissioned by the DHSS. We would have been unable to produce as much without the blessing of the Research Committee of the Association of Directors of Social Services, and the co-operation of the managers of the agencies which have provided us with material. Those from the agencies who wrote the accounts should be considered co-authors. Howard Glennerster and Adrian Webb made valuable comments as the external examiners for the first author's doctoral thesis based on this project. At the PSSRU, Andrew Bebbington and Man-Sum Tong provided statistical advice and customised software. Anita Whitley and Anne Walker typed the text and the many tables of volume II with unfailing humour and skill. Jane Dennett and Nick Brawn have brought their usual energy to the task of preparing the discs for publication and reminding the impatient authors of what remained to be done before it could be despatched. At Gower, Sarah Sutton has dealt with publication in the way which we have come to expect of the handling of this Unit's series.

Bleddyn Davies
July 1988

1 The Production of Welfare and Efficiency-Improving Innovation

The Innovatory Imperative

It is commonly argued that the welfare state is faced both by increased demand and a decreased growth rate with which to meet that demand. Such pressure is certainly acutely felt in the health and personal social services budget, which is faced with the resource consequences of an ageing population, escalating unit costs of institutional care, and historically decreasing growth rates.

One possible but demanding response would be to increase the efficiency with which existing resources are deployed so as to secure more output from the same budget. In particular, a long-standing objective of health and personal social services policy has been the promotion of modal shift so as to provide relatively less of expensive hospital and residential care and relatively more of community-based care. Such forms of care, it is argued, are often cheaper, better, and desired by clients themselves. With the arrival of a more financially constrained policy climate from the mid-1970s onwards, this objective has been pursued by new central mechanisms such as joint finance and the Care in the Community programme. Local government has produced other responses through its own initiative. Yet at the same time there is dissatisfaction with the pace of change: many of the issues of the 1980s have been prominent since the 1950s and have proved to be enduring problems.

Thus a central problem over these three decades has been one of a *continuing gap in innovations* (or failure to achieve change in service systems) in the community care for elderly people. It is of course hard to imagine that large-scale, public sector bureaucracies would take readily to the implementation of efficiency-improving innovation as a response to fiscal pressure. This leads to two dangers in relying on such an innovatory strategy. The first is that form may take over from content: too often the cult of the new results in innovation being valued as a good in itself rather than as a means to achieving 'better' services. The second is the underestimation of the obstacles to change in bureaucracies given that radical innovation may be organisationally impossible or at least extremely difficult to implement. The best may here become the enemy of the good, if time and effort spent on the design of failed innovations could have been put into the less exciting task of delivering good basic services.

The innovatory option is by no means an easy one. But if service systems are to achieve qualitative transformation which goes beyond purely incremental change, then it will be precisely through such processes of innovation. In order to assess the potential advantages and disadvantages associated with these incremental and innovatory change strategies, there is a need to study the process of innovation in the health and personal social services in some detail.

In this book, such processes of innovation are specifically examined in the care of elderly people. 'Innovation' is defined as a change in the product or service offered by the adopting organisation. As such it can be distinguished from 'change' or the re-allocation of resources between established budgetary heads. Innovation in the community care of elderly people might be expected to secure a substantial return for the providing agencies because the elderly are major consumers of resources. As far as health and personal social services expenditure is concerned, the over-75s consume nearly five times the resources per head as the population as a whole (Cmnd 8494-ii, 1982, p.42). With specific reference to the personal social services budget, just one service — residential care for elderly people (Part III) — accounted for 23 per cent of gross current expenditure in 1982–83. In addition the unit cost of Part III rose by more than 10 per cent in constant prices between 1976–77 and 1982–83 (House of Commons Select Committee on the Social Services, 1984, HCP 395-i, pp.14–16), placing even greater pressure on the residential care budget. Demographic pressures continue to be considerable. The percentage of the population aged 65 or over increased from 11.7 per cent in 1961 to 15.2 in 1981 (Central Statistical Office, 1984, p.18). Although the number of 65 to 75 year olds is now likely to reach a plateau, and marginally declined between 1981 and 1984, this is offset by a continuing increase in the numbers of the very elderly whose resource

9

consumption is highest. So resource pressures and demographic trends continue to make innovation in services for elderly people an area of strategic importance. A major problem has, however, been the failure to generate a critical perspective which gets beyond the use of 'innovation' as a positive and value-laden term. The next section argues that the concept of 'efficiency improvement' offers one way forward.

A Production of Welfare Perspective

We lay stress on the need for a more analytic approach in the examination of innovations. This is because a purely rhetorical commitment to innovation as a good in itself — as the outward and visible mark of high-achieving management — may be elevated above a consideration of its effects on service delivery. Additionally, innovators may be pursuing private agendas, in conflict with formally sanctioned goals. Since innovation is only desirable if it results in 'better' services, it is necessary to derive indicators against which the impact of innovation can be assessed. The production of welfare perspective provides one way of doing this, centred on securing the optimal use of scarce resources.

There are various reasons for supposing that the use of such resources will be non-optimal. Human service agencies produce goods paid for out of taxation and free at the point of delivery and may thus become insensitive both to the needs of consumers and the development of efficient and equitable rationing systems. Such agencies may be areal monopolists able to impose or withhold consumption or serving captive, low-income clients who have little recourse to private markets (as with many elderly clients). Although the maximand is formally assumed to be the reduction of need rather than the pursuit of profit, individual actors will have their own objectives. There are other limitations on the action of human service organisations: they are constrained by statute, by central government intervention and more diffusely by informed climates of opinion. Innovation is here unlikely to emerge through the sudden technological push seen in sunrise industries (what is the human service organisation equivalent of the digital watch?), but through a gradual change in the stock of social knowledge or an incremental widening of the legislative basis of legitimate action.

Despite these circumstances, a production of welfare model nevertheless retains validity. Human service organisations exist to provide services, that is to transform resources into outputs which produce enhanced outcomes for clients. Where there is discretion over service allocation (and departments vary substantially in the proportion of the budget for elderly people devoted to residential or community services), then such agencies are in an analogous position to a multi-product firm which seeks not only technical efficiency in each production process but also allocative efficiency in the balance of outputs produced. Especially when there is fiscal pressure, there will be a requirement to produce the best mix of outputs at least cost.

In the production of welfare perspective, concepts of *input* and *output* and of the relationship between them are basic conceptual building blocks. Inputs can be divided into the conventional factors of production, *resource inputs* and *non-resource inputs* which are not physical (such as regime or style of organisation). It is important to note that the input/output relationship may be pervasively affected by key non-resource inputs, such as mode of organisation, practice style and level of staff motivation. So although baseline and inno-vatory services might cost exactly the same amount to the agency, there may still be wide variation in the level of output (client welfare gain) achieved.

The concept of output can also be disaggregated. *Final output* can be defined as the difference between the well-being observed after a caring intervention compared with the level of well-being in the absence of a caring intervention (Knapp, 1984, p.31). In many cases, however, final output information will not be available as few agencies routinely build in evaluation of their programmes. Secondly, many organisations will simplify their search routines for new technologies, confining them to a comparison between a few 'off-the-shelf' alterna-tives rather than engaging in developmental work based on examin-ation of final outputs. Interest may therefore also centre on *inter-mediate outputs*. These are defined 'in terms of the care services themselves, rather than the effects of these services on the clients. Intermediate outputs will thus be expressed in terms of levels of provision, throughput and quality of care. They are indicators of performance, service or activity rather than indicators of effect, influ-ence or impact' (Knapp, 1984, p.32).

Intermediate output indicators closely resemble the process evalu-ations which have emerged in the American health services approach to quality assurance (Donabedian, 1982) which aim at producing measures of service processes which are explicit and precise enough to permit evaluative judgement. Chapter 2 will follow this approach in developing measures for the process evaluation of innovatory schemes.

Efficiency Improvement

The term 'efficiency improvement' is particularly difficult to conceptualise in human service organisations where there are no consumer or market tests, but Davies and Challis (1986) suggest that the term can be usefully broken down into five dimensions:

(i) *horizontal target efficiency* (the extent to which those deemed to need a service receive it);

(ii) *vertical target efficiency* (the extent to which those who receive a service need it);

(iii) *input mix efficiency* (the extent to which the input mix is adjusted to relative prices and constraints in supply);

(iv) *market efficiency* (the extent to which the mix of outputs produced reflects valuations); and

(v) *technical efficiency* (the degree to which a given combination of resources is deployed to maximise outputs).

Innovations may contribute to none, some or all of these dimensions. Although (iii) has been a long-standing objective of both national and local policy, there is a major link between (iii) and (iv), which suggests an output-centred approach to the definition of efficiency. Modal shift towards community care implies the redesigning of services so as to improve ability to care for clients at higher dependency levels. Let us consider each of these dimensions in turn.

Horizontal target efficiency

More successful case-finding activity has been a long-standing preoccupation of agencies from the creation of 'one door on which to knock' following the Seebohm Report (Cmnd 3703, 1968), through the needs surveys of the early 1970s to the renewed interest in interweaving with the informal sector apparent in the Barclay Report (1982). Different case-finding issues arise for mainstream services and special projects. The former often pursue enhanced case finding by means such as the attachment of a social worker to medical settings which do not necessitate service innovation. However, Hadley and McGrath (1984) seek to promote case finding through changes in the role and style of fieldwork teams so as to blur the boundary with the local community. The adoption of patch-style working has, if taken seriously, important implications for the ways in which fieldwork and domiciliary services are delivered. For special projects, case finding is a far more immediate issue and many innovations will engage in promotional activity as a means of stimulating referrals from sometimes wary service providers. However, direct outreach to potential clients is less likely, so case-finding activity may proceed without pervasive changes in roles and the style of operation of the innovatory scheme.

Vertical target efficiency

Vertical target efficiency refers to the degree to which service resources are devoted to those who are deemed to be in need. Poor vertical targeting results in a situation where supply creates its own demand, with little thought being given to the objectives of intervention. A common criticism of the home help service has been that expansionist momentum has prevented the clear setting of aims and objectives. Social work with elderly people in many areas has consisted of routine visiting of large caseloads on a 'monitoring' basis, rather than task-centred casework. Better programme targeting may either take the non-innovatory form of issuing policy guidelines for existing services or the innovatory design of services targeted at particular subgroups. At the level of the individual, better targeting can proceed through the introduction of holistic and problem-based assessment rather than assessment for eligibility for discrete services.

Input mix efficiency

Input mix efficiency refers to the choice between service modes, bearing in mind relative prices and constraints on supply. The further development of community care in response to the distinct cost hierarchy observable between hospital, residential and community based modes of care (Tinker, 1984; Audit Commission, 1985) and the increasing pressure on the institutional care sector has formed a dominant theme of policy at national and increasingly at local level. Within the hospital sector the number of geriatric beds has been held steady despite increased numbers of elderly people (from about 5 million in 1953 to 7 million in 1983), whereas turnover and outpatients work have increased.

The knock-on pressure from the hospital sector was originally met through the expansion of local authority residential care, but from the mid-1970s onwards tighter constraints on local authority expenditure, especially on the capital side, made this policy less viable.

An increased policy stress on community care was evident as early as the mid-1950s (Boucher, 1957; Ministry of Health, 1957) and included backing for acutely oriented specialist geriatric medicine, a stress on greater co-operation between hospitals and Part III establishments and the definition of appropriate eligibility criteria, and expansion of community care alternatives to residential provision. These themes were to recur. Indeed many of the domiciliary care 'innovations' launched in the 1980s seem identical to those commended in the Annual Reports of the Ministry of Health 30 years earlier. Most of the strategic issues facing social services departments (SSDs) in the provision of support for their most resource-consuming client group have been evident for a similar period (Davies, 1981b). Input mix substitution was often seen in crude terms as a choice between defined modes of care. The setting of protected indicative growth rates for community services was a major theme of the *Priorities* document (DHSS, 1976a), but the qualitative transformation of such services in response to rising levels of dependency was not explored. While the dominant input mix substitution objective has in the past been narrowly defined as shifting the balance of care between and within two public agencies (the National Health Service — NHS — and SSDs), there is no reason to suppose that this agenda is fixed. A new input substitution question is the expansion of publicly financed private residential care which has reversed the modal shift to community care.

Output mix efficiency

The danger of a narrow focus on input substitution is that no thought will be given to the output mix efficiency of community services, that is the extent to which they reflect valuations. Where full evaluative information on the effects of service provision on client well-being is not available (that is, in many cases), proxy measures of service process will have to be used. Such quality assessment is a judgement concerning the process of care, based on the extent to which that care is thought to be associated with valued outcomes.

The derivation of such process measures can be related to a theory of client need and of requisite service response. Isaacs and Neville (1976) distinguish between three need categories, based on the interval between necessary episodes of help. Thus 'long interval' (often domestic care) needs require care tasks once every 24 hours or less often. The exact time when these tasks is performed is unimportant and no special skill is required of the helper. For other clients, with 'short interval' needs, basic tasks (often personal care tasks) must be performed every few hours each day, although help does not have to be provided at an exact time and no special skill is required of the helper. 'Critical interval' needs arise at short and unpredictable intervals requiring continuously present, skilful and acceptable help. Incontinence of urine or faeces, dementia and a tendency to fall are examples of such critical interval need. Isaacs and Neville (1976)

14

further distinguished between the needs of elderly people by measuring the degree of solitude or the period of the day during which the elderly person is left alone.

In order to respond to higher levels of need, community care services can move along two dimensions. The first consists of enhanced *service content*, especially the performance of personal care tasks at specific times or outside normal working hours (such as getting up and putting to bed, feeding and toileting). The other dimension is *case management* or the performance of such tasks as assessment, the negotiation, planning and arrangement of a care plan tailored to circumstances which fills client deficits, and monitoring the success of a care plan and adapting it as needed (Davies and Challis, 1986). The better construction of care plans which move beyond the assessment of eligibility for particular services is likely to produce such 'signs and symptoms' of efficiency improvement as problem-based assessments, key workers, case conferences and liaison with other service providers. The construction of daily care plans is especially important for those with critical interval needs (such as the demented) who cannot be left unsupported for long periods.

Technical efficiency

Technical efficiency reflects the extent to which output is maximised within a given service. Often moves to improve technical innovation may not involve service innovation, such as attempts to rationalise home help mileage. In other areas the introduction of new technology will provide an opportunity for service innovation aimed at improving technical efficiency. For example, the Audit Commission (1985) suggests that revenue savings could be achieved in the meals-on-wheels service by a move to a cook-chill system, if necessary combined with the purchase of ovens and freezers for recipients.

Study Design and Method

Alternative approaches

Studies of organisations are often divided into two main types, with important implications for the method adopted. *Deductive* studies (Weeks, 1973) are likely to display the following assumptions: (i) that the structural and functional similarities of organisations are more important than the cultural differences between organisations; (ii) that the overall social context within which organisations develop is more important than the particular development of each organisation; (iii) that there exists a logic of organisational functioning related to the achievement of goals; and (iv) that management control is effectively achieved by the implementation of formal rules. By contrast the inductive approach to organisational analysis asserts: (i) that the processual aspects of organisations are more important than their formal structure; (ii) that informally generated meanings are the real basis of organisational control; and (iii) that motivation varies according to context.

The study of innovation has usually been conducted in an inductive manner, concentrating on case study analysis which explores the historical and informal organisational context (Donnison, Chapman, Meacher, Sears and Urwin, 1975; Glennerster, Korman, Marslen-Wilson and Meredith, 1982). The advantage of an inductive approach is the generation of deep knowledge of the ways in which schemes function in practice and deviate from more formal rationales (often provided by senior management). The disadvantage of inductive analysis lies in the difficulty in generalising or engaging in comparative analysis, for which a larger number of observations are needed. First, the need to develop low-level generalisation must be considered. American writers such as Aiken and Hage (1971) have by contrast adopted a more deductive approach, attempting quantitatively to predict the propensity to innovate (defined simply as the average number of 'innovations' launched per year) through measures of formal organisational structure. As a result of such analysis they were able to lend empirical support in a human service organisation context to the more general argument that the organic organisation has many characteristics which facilitate innovation. Boaden (1971) used similar techniques in predicting the propensity of English local government agencies to innovate. Second, there is a need to develop comparative analysis across schemes as well as across organisations. Too often the precise service content of innovations is not considered, due to greater interest in the identification of those organisational characteristics which facilitate innovation. Yet it may be possible to identify broad groupings of schemes which differ from each other in their lines of development. The development of a comparative typology of schemes requires of course a large number of observations. The cost of the deductive approach lies in the loss of understanding of how a small number of schemes actually operate.

Study method

As our interest lay in attempts to generalise about organisational behaviour and to plot a typology of schemes, a decision was made to go for less information about more schemes, rather than more information about a smaller number of schemes. The basic method was the postal trawl for information. An initial letter was sent out to all SSDs, health districts and housing departments in England and Wales, as well as a small number of selected voluntary organisations (such as Age Concern and MIND). Follow-up telephone calls were made if necessary, as were a small number of site visits where possible. It was not, however, possible to conduct a systematic quality control exercise. The raw responses were catalogued in Ferlie (1982). The information returned was then coded on the basis of the process indicators contained in Chapter 2 (Ferlie, Challis and Davies, 1983).

Although postal trawls are one means of gathering basic information across a large number of sites, they pose some methodological difficulties. The first is the possibility of a poor or variable response rate. As we worked from a Unit which concentrated on the personal social services, there was obviously a possibility that the contacts we had built up in that field would mean a higher response rate from SSDs than other agencies. Table 1.1 indicates that while a satisfactory response rate was indeed obtained from SSDs, in the other sectors response was much lower. While sufficient observations were obtained in the SSD sector to permit modelling work, this was not possible in the housing and health fields.

A second difficulty consisted of the loss of control over the information returned, which varied substantially in both quantity and quality. Although follow-up phone calls improved the quality of information in some cases, in others lines of communication between HQ-based respondents and schemes in the areas were too poor to produce more information. We have had to assume that if we have been told about it, it exists and that if we have not been told about it, it does not exist. In some authorities, liaison officers circulated our request

Table 1.1
Response rate

	Population*	Sample	%
Social services departments	116	70	60
Housing departments	403	14	4
Health districts	201	28	14

Note
*   England and Wales (1983).
Source: Ferlie (1982).

for information widely, while in others only information routinely available to the centre was returned. Few respondents followed the checklist of points supplied. Nevertheless a substantial body of information was returned on over 200 schemes which was sufficient for comparative work, enabling analysis to proceed beyond the case-study approach dominant within British social policy.

We have thus argued that the development of innovation in services for elderly people is now of strategic significance for social care agencies and that the analysis of such innovations is best pursued from an efficiency perspective. Different dimensions of efficiency were distinguished. We outlined the rationale for adopting postally-based instruments as a means of generating comparative analysis.

We now turn to our development of process indicators of efficiency improvement which were used as a coding framework for the mass of returned material.

2 Process Measures of Efficiency Improvement

In this chapter we consider the formulation of proxy process-based measures of efficiency improvement. As the regulation of the private sector did not emerge as a major theme in the data base, other aspects of this quality assurance literature (such as the assessment and securing of compliance) need not be reviewed at this stage. The formulation of appropriate standards is by no means a simple task. Writing in a residential care context, Davies (1986) argues such standards should be:

- specific requirements, not vague injunctions;
- feasible for providers to achieve;
- assessable by a regulatory agency;
- able to yield evidence of non compliance hard enough to stand up in the enforcement process;
- covering features of greatest importance to the entire range of interested parties, including residents, relatives, agencies financing care and pressure groups concerned with equity issues; and
- as much as possible, defined in terms of inputs, processes and outcomes of direct evaluative significance in their own right.

Present-day regulatory frameworks are much more primitive. The American guidelines for the regulation of private sector residential care demanded paper compliance on management and resource issues rather than evidence of compliance on patient care issues (Davies,

1986). The British regulatory framework (Challis, 1985) focuses on physical standards (such as fire precautions) rather than the quality of care. However, alternative frameworks are available and will now be considered.

Previous Approaches to Process Evaluation

Evaluation through explicit process criteria is prominent in the American health as well as residential care context, where legislation, notably the 1972 amendments to the Social Security Acts, mandated the formation of Professional Standards Review Organizations (PSROs) as a response both to escalation of the costs of medical care and concern about poor standards of publicly-financed care. Fears that PSROs were counterproductive, in encouraging professionals to overprescribe, led to their repeal in 1982, although they were recreated as Professional Review Organizations (PROs) through the Peer Improvement Act of 1982. Physicians remained the group with primary responsibility for review, although there has recently been an increased role for utilisation review (rather than peer review) by fiscal intermediaries (Baker, 1983). The PSRO approach made it possible to consider the performance of professionals against indicators of 'good' behaviour, usually within a peer review context. In contrast, PROs place more emphasis on cost-related criteria, in response to the criticism that PSROs had themselves proved cost-ineffective (Congressional Budget Office, 1981). Associated with the rapid development of the requirement for evaluation has been the emergence of a process literature designed to tackle the methodological problems thrown up.

'Quality assessment' represents a key concept within this literature. Donabedian's work on process measures in health care defines 'quality' in the following terms: 'an assessment of quality is a judgement concerning the process of care, based on the extent to which that care contributes to valued outcomes' (Donabedian, 1982, p.3).

The criteria used for the assessment of quality can be broken down into three different domains. 'Structure' refers to the resources used in the provision of care, 'process' refers to the activities that constitute care and 'outcomes' are the consequences to health (ibid, p.6). The development of process criteria represents a major element of Donabedian's work. To be of use such criteria should aim at a degree of high specification with a detailed operationalisation which permits measurement. There is also the question of how such criteria can be best derived. One method is to rely on a panel of 'experts', although the links between professional judgement and outcome criteria may

20

be tenuous. The other method (which was adopted in this study) is to rely on a literature survey, although this also entails difficulties. The literature may be very partial in coverage or poorly relate process to outcome measurements.

Process criteria (ibid, p.362) can include elements based on the control of costs as well as elements relating to the quality of care. Thus justification of admission, of continued stay and the use of cost benchmarks form important elements of the *efficiency* dimension. The *effectiveness* dimension is explored through the use of indicators such as verification of the diagnosis, the performance of diagnostic and therapeutic procedures required by this diagnosis, the avoidance of service underutilisation and liaison with family and community where this is relevant. As quality assessment methods have developed, so cost and efficiency analysis have assumed greater importance than in the initial professionally-dominated peer review contexts which concentrated on issues of programme effectiveness.

Signs and Symptoms of Efficiency

This study was based on a similar design. Organisations were asked to supply information organised around a set of common heads. Further details were obtained through follow-up telephone calls where necessary. This information was then subjected to a contents analysis on the basis of explicit process criteria, to produce a data base for later analysis.

There were two main dimensions to the process framework developed for the content analysis of the returned mass of material. The first was the extent to which each process sign could be seen as contributing to the five definitions of efficiency identified in Chapter 1. To recapitulate, 'horizontal target efficiency' can be defined as the extent to which persons for whom a mode of intervention is the most cost-effective receive it. 'Vertical target efficiency' is the extent to which a mode's resources are allocated to those who are most cost-effectively helped by it. 'Market efficiency' is the extent to which output mix is consistent with relative valuation of outputs. 'Input mix efficiency' is measured by the degree to which the input mix reflects prices and supply so as to maximise outputs. 'Technical efficiency' reflects the extent to which given resources are deployed so as to maximise outputs (Davies and Challis, 1986).

A second question is whether schemes which most increase efficiency are more likely to emerge within specific organisational contexts. Schemes display differential attrition rates over time: they may develop into major resources, or remain marginal to the mainstream pattern of service provision. This dimension therefore concerns *organisational process*. The next section will outline how each of these dimensions was broken down and operationalised. This classification in turn formed the basis for coding frames for the different sectors of care. This chapter explains why those coding frames were built up as they were.

So each sign is directly related to the efficiency argument. But in addition there is a second efficiency-related distinction to be drawn between signs which contribute to case management and those which contribute to service content. The production of welfare perspective argues that case management can be broken down into a number of core tasks which are performed along the natural history of the case. The essential tasks of case management fall into five main stages: definition of appropriate populations, case finding, assessment, care packaging and monitoring. Each stage is considered in turn. But in addition the content of the services packaged needs to be considered and may be enhanced in a number of ways. The argument is summarised in Table 2.1 which lists the signs chosen, their focus on the stages of case management or enhanced service content and their likely contribution to efficiency.

Each stage of case management and aspect of service content is now discussed in turn.

Definition of appropriate populations

Targeting by eligibility criteria At the level of the individual, assessment represents a mechanism for achieving vertical target efficiency. This may be complemented at programme level by efforts to improve targeting on subgroups. The danger of poor vertically targeted services is that resources will be spread too thinly, leading to a shallow gradient in service allocation in respect of need and a failure to achieve priority objectives.

There are a number of eligibility criteria which could be associated with attempts to develop better targeted services. Clients on the margin of dependency between that requiring community and requiring institutional care represent a high 'pay off' area for developing community-based services, although the precise nature of such margins will vary from one system to another. Concern has repeatedly been expressed about the failure to co-ordinate care associated with the transfer of cases from hospital to SSD agencies (Amos, 1973) or indeed from SSD residential to domiciliary care. The need for some clients of marginal dependency to enter Part III might be avoided by concerted earlier action. On the basis of a study of admissions to Part III in a London Borough, Sinclair, Levin, Neill, Gorbach and Williams

Table 2.1
**Process signs, case management, and service
content and efficiency**

Sign	Case management or service content	Aspect of efficiency
Targeting (eligibility criteria)	Case management: defines appropriate population	Vertical target
Targeting (client subgroup)	Case management: defines appropriate population	Vertical target
	Service content: variety	Output mix
Vertical targeting	Case management: defines appropriate population	Vertical target
Horizontal targeting	Case management: case finding	Horizontal target
Assessment	Case management: assessment	Output mix
Care packaging	Case management: care packaging	Output mix
	gap filling	Input mix
Service arranging	Case management: care packaging	Output mix
		Input mix
Monitoring	Case management: monitoring	Output mix
		Input mix
Key worker	Case management: care packaging	Output mix
		Input mix
Direct work	Service content	Output mix
		Technical
Service variety and flexibility	Service content	Output mix
		Technical
Short-term service	Service content	Technical
Rehabilitation	Service content	Technical
Lower-cost mode	Case management and service content	Input mix
Informal carer support	Case management and service content	Input mix
Production function	Service content	Technical
Source of finance	Case management and service content	Input mix

(1986) argue that the admission of about a third of applicants could have been avoided by action at the point of application, and that of another third by earlier action.

A second criterion could be to concentrate provision on elderly clients who lack informal carers in order to manage vulnerable elderly people in the community. Thus Sinclair et al. (1986) also report that Part III applicants were more likely to be living on their own than elderly people of similar age in the community and much less likely to be currently married. These findings about the social unrepresentativeness of Part III admissions were endorsed by Willcocks, Peace and Kellaher (1982). Thirdly, some geriatricians adopt an age-related admissions policy (such as 70 or 75) in order to concentrate on cases where geriatric forms of pathology are most evident.

Targeting by client subgroup Programmes may be targeted not only by eligibility criteria but by subgroup criteria which enable target clienteles to be more tightly drawn. But there is also a service content argument which affects the degree of market efficiency. As different needs require different services, only where there is requisite service variety will it be possible to match resources to needs, rather than the other way round. Both social work and domiciliary care for elderly people have traditionally exhibited little service variation and have failed to reflect the different patterns of need presented. Thus social work with the elderly (Goldberg, Mortimer and Williams, 1970) has often been seen as consisting of routine and undemanding requests for practical services that could safely be left to social work assistants. In the case of the home help service, Hedley and Norman (1982) illustrate the very recent origins of specialist personal care home help schemes targeted at the more dependent elderly.

Targeting services by client subgroup represents another way in which services could be made more vertically target efficient. For example, dementing elderly (80 per cent of whom are cared for at home) will present special needs. Levin, Sinclair and Gorbach's study (1982) of demented elderly at home assessed the dementia as moderate in 35 per cent of cases and as severe in 42 per cent of cases. They add:

> The diagnosis of dementia and usually its degree was correlated with such problems as falls, incontinence, repetition, restlessness, mistaking the supporters for others, dangerous/risky acts, lack of purposeful activity, hitting out at the supporters, disturbing the supporters' sleep and inability to carry on normal everyday conversations (ibid, p.232).

Conventional thin-spread inputs are likely to be less market efficient in the management of dementia than special services which emphasise such case management features as early identification, multidisciplinary assessment (medical and social), care packaging, support for

24

relatives and follow-up. In addition the content of back-up services can also be improved. Specialist home help services for the demented have emerged in a few areas, such as North Buckinghamshire (Hedley and Norman, 1982, p.33) where 60 specially recruited and trained home helps offer a service (including during anti-social hours) to elderly people referred from a Department of Mental Health for the Elderly.

Challis and Davies (1986) discuss the special requirements of social work with the dementing including the need to *care pattern* or build a regular pattern of care based on the memory strengths retained by the elderly client, focusing on the pattern of coping as a whole (rather than accepting the obvious problems mentioned at referral) and responding to that through comprehensive and flexible case management.

The provision of services for the demented represents only one aspect of client subgroup targeting. Other elderly subgroups which exhibit special needs include stroke victims, the incontinent, the socially isolated, the deaf and the blind, the rootless, the physically handicapped, the bereaved, those at risk of falling and of course stressed informal carers of elderly people. Full targeting requires the development of expertise with all these subgroups. In some cases, the development of subgroup expertise will be formally built into the design of an innovation from the beginning. In other schemes, specialist expertise may build up gradually, as a response to unanticipated referral patterns, and hence subgroup targeting may sometimes emerge informally.

Vertical targeting Vertical target efficiency refers to the degree to which service resources are devoted to those who most benefit from them. Targeting exercises at programme level have already been considered, but these can be complemented by vertical targeting within programmes. Evidence suggests that there is poor vertical targeting at client level in a number of services. In the case of the home help service, local studies have found little relationship between levels of need and service allocation (Gwynne and Fean, 1978; Hurley and Wolstenholme, 1980). Nor does growth appear to lead automatically to better vertical targeting; the Devon study by Howell, Boldy and Smith (1979) suggested that a more favourable balance of resources to needs did not lead to a steeper gradient in the allocation of service. Hurley and Wolstenholme (1980) found that home helps were frequently undertaking such tasks as dusting which clients were capable of doing themselves. Bebbington's comparison (1979) of 1962 and 1976 data sets suggested that the home help service, although it had expanded, had become more thinly spread over a larger number of clients. This argument was confirmed by Hedley and Norman (1982) who estimate that the average number of hours per case fell from 4.7 in 1967 to 2.09 in 1979.

The meals service also exhibits low vertical target efficiency at individual level. A Kent study (Brotherton, 1975) found 40 per cent of recipients cooking for themselves on days when meals were not delivered. The study by Johnson, di Gregorio and Harrison (1981) concluded that very few of those in receipt of the meals service were in need of a nutritional supplement or at nutritional risk. Central guidelines were outlined in Circular 5/70 (DHSS, 1970) which suggested targeting on those living alone or who had difficulty in preparing a main meal, those in temporary difficulty and those with inadequate cooking facilities or poor motivation who could not get meals from other sources. However, Means (1981) found little evidence of such targeting in at least some of his case study authorities. The corollary is that intensive help is not provided. Often meals will be available only twice a week or in term time. Some authorities are now arguing the case for better vertical targeting of the meals service: Bedfordshire SSD (1978) states that meals should only be provided to those most in need for between five and seven days a week.

Case finding

Horizontal targeting Horizontal target efficiency (Bebbington and Davies, 1983) refers to the extent to which persons for whom a mode of intervention is the most appropriate receive it. There are grounds for supposing that a substantial degree of horizontal target inefficiency exists in mainstream services. Bebbington and Davies (1983) produce evidence to show a higher degree of horizontal target efficiency than vertical target efficiency in the home help service: unmet need was more of a problem than the allocation of service to those with low dependency levels. In residential care the silting-up of places and thus difficulties in securing admission is encouraged by the historic lack of emphasis on short-term beds, although the number of short-term beds has recently expanded (Allen, 1982). Horizontal target inefficiency may have particularly pernicious effects in the care of elderly people because of the 'spiral of decline'. Primary prevention is a hallmark of acute geriatrics (Evans, 1981) and is paralleled by the emphasis on secondary prevention in patch-based schemes (Hadley and McGrath, 1984).

Securing an adequate number of referrals is a problem frequently encountered by innovatory schemes. There are a number of ways in which schemes can promote horizontal target efficiency. First, steps can be taken to increase the uptake of services either by introducing

26

new forms of service which reduce silting-up, by removing charges, or by introducing more locally accessible services. In some cases new schemes which have been introduced on a charging basis have reported problems in generating adequate uptake. Other means of increasing uptake include the use of community alarm, warden or street warden systems, whether statutory or voluntary, acting as a form of preventive surveillance. In primary care, the unreported pathology evident in the elderly client group has long been evident (Williamson, Stokoe, Gray, Fisher, Smith, Maghee and Stephenson, 1964). Screening exercises designed to identify incipient and remediable pathology form a common focus of development in this setting. Another mechanism whereby uptake can be increased is through improved or automatic referral procedures. Assessments may be mandatory for all patients coming off a ward, or special arrangements may be negotiated for referral transfer between, say, the home help and community nursing services.

Assessment, care planning and monitoring

Assessment Moving on now to discuss assessment and care planning, a different set of efficiency arguments will be introduced. In order to achieve output mix efficiency, it is important to match resources to needs and not vice versa. One should think first about ends and then go on to consider available means, doing this in the least constrained form possible. The assessment task consists of the identification of needs and hence the specification of ends, while care packaging consists of the elaboration of means to meet those ends. Assessment thus centres on the identification of welfare shortfalls as legitimated targets for intervention and is a necessary precondition for ensuring output mix efficiency. Goldberg, Mortimer and Williams (1970) found that such diagnostic thinking was associated with professional training and that trained social workers were more likely than untrained workers to recognise signs of depression (apathy, loss of appetite), of family stress or of an unreasonable burden placed on informal carers. Traditionally social work with elderly people is carried out by staff who are on the lower grades, carry larger caseloads, and lack qualifications (Holme and Maizels, 1978). The destructive impact of large caseloads on time available for assessment may be severe.

Often assessment skills have remained at a low level. Vickery (1981) found that effective social work with elderly people was obstructed by primitive assessment procedures: needs were seen in terms of means (specific services) rather than ends (welfare shortfalls), there was little allocative control over key resources, and little account taken of informal and neighbourhood inputs.

27

Recent developments in assessment instrumentation reflect attempts to be more explicit about means and ends in social interventions. The instrumentation described by Goldberg and Warburton (1979) was designed in order to achieve such goals. The Thanet Community Care Project (Challis and Davies, 1986; Davies and Challis, 1986) designed assessment instrumentation covering the key domains of household structure, the health and needs of principal carers, physical and mental health status, difficulties in activities of daily living, and financial and housing circumstances as a means of identifying key welfare shortfalls. Challis and Davies define the assessment process in the following terms:

> Thus the function of assessment was not to ask the question all too commonly formulated in the care of elderly people — namely, 'what service does this elderly person require?', but rather to pose two separate questions: first, 'what difficulties are this elderly person and their carers experiencing?' and secondly, 'what is the most appropriate means of dealing with these difficulties?' (1986, p.46).

Less ambitious attempts to improve assessment procedures have also been implemented for more limited purposes. Some authorities (Ferlie, 1982) have introduced standardised assessment scales, usually to measure physical dependency. Assessment centres concentrate on the examination of the needs of the elderly client. Some community-orientated psychogeriatric units emphasise domiciliary assessments and use attached social workers to carry out social background reports, including a consideration of the needs of relatives. Pointers to consider in evaluating the quality of assessment procedures include the grade of the staff allocated the work, and the number and level of resources over which the assessors have control. There is little incentive for staff to carry out detailed and time-consuming assessments if they cannot be related to available resources. Multidisciplinary assessment will also be important where there is a mixture of social and medical needs. However, many innovations (Ferlie, 1982) report no increase in the breadth of the assessment process, no multidisciplinary involvement, and no stress on casework skills. Compared with assessment procedures in the care of mentally handicapped children (M. Plank, 1982), few report the close involvement of informal carers in the assessment process, let alone the client. Improved assessment procedures represent an important area for development.

Arranging a care package Whereas the assessment task is based on an examination of ends, care packaging activity reflects an interest in means. It contributes to market efficiency through its implementation of the assessment judgement. Although the indirect role of social workers in care packaging was acknowledged in the Barclay Report (1982) and becomes even more important in increasingly differentiated service systems, there is insufficient awareness of the skill level required. Thus Goldberg, Mortimer and Williams (1970) found that trained social workers were able to provide more resources for their elderly clients than untrained social workers, despite their extra emphasis on direct work tasks. This was because their repertoire of intervention techniques was greater and they were able to tap more formal and informal resources. They also comment:

> Collaboration with a host of other statutory and voluntary agencies on behalf of the elderly client, acting as a co-ordinator of these services, ensuring that they function smoothly and appropriately, emerged as a central task in the present fragmented personal social services for the aged (Goldberg, Mortimer and Williams, 1970, p.197).

If care packaging is to go beyond routine administrative activity, attention should be directed to such techniques as enabling, the creation as well as the mobilisation of resources, and integration of service allocation with cost information. Enabling can be seen as an aspect of market efficiency. The use of cost information in care packaging contributes to input mix efficiency (the achievement of welfare objectives identified by the assessment process through constructing cost-effective service packages, which may vary in their nature from one local system to another). Input mix efficiency is also achieved through the mobilisation of informal resources which can fill the gaps left by the public sector support system.

These signs can be considered in turn. First, a social worker will often have to 'enable' clients to receive services, given anxieties about loss of autonomy. Enabling may also take place through interweaving with informal carers, so as to reduce the level of strain to acceptable limits, to enable carers to tolerate a degree of risk and to avoid overprotective behaviour. Effective interweaving is contingent on a good knowledge of the informal caring network, yet Bayley and Parker (1980) found that social workers have little such knowledge (when compared with home helps and wardens). Second, social workers may create as well as mobilise resources, especially informal, neighbourhood or voluntary resources. The balance of such resources will vary substantially from one area to another. Thus Walker (1975) argues that urban networks are based on kinship with a secondary role for friends, while rural networks accord more importance to friends and neighbours. The balance of formal resources will also vary from one service system to another, indicating the important role of small area variations in determining optimal methods of care packaging. A further source of complexity in care packaging is the multiple needs of many elderly people, including physical dependency, social isolation and mental impairment. In the case of dementing elderly people, care packaging will be necessary to establish a round-the-clock support system which could manage periods of risk. A final point relates to the integration of service allocation with cost information. This may be dependent on the delegation of power to case managers who are themselves then held responsible as decentralised cost centres working within total budgets with shadow price information.

So care packaging will vary along two dimensions. First there is the tightness of the specification of the care packaging method. The commitment may be very general, or may include specific interest in tailoring to individual needs or providing informal carer support. High quality care packaging will also be sensitive to the costs of the various services being packaged, as often allocators prescribe services in the absence of cost information. Secondly, care packaging will vary according to the range of services packaged. Some schemes will restrict themselves to negotiating internal SSD resources, whereas others will focus on external agencies or create new sources of care.

Service arranging Basic care packaging is dependent on good working relationships between agencies. However, where relations are bad, care packaging will be difficult to achieve informally. Output and input mix inefficiency could both arise because of this. One response to this danger is to set up formal negotiating procedures to process requests for service allocation. More importantly, the construction of care plans may be dependent on changes in the line of executive authority so that front-line staff have greater control over the allocation of services. In the home help service, Hey (1980) describes the emergent role of social services officer in which home help organisers directly allocate a number of basic services. Such developments in social work were commended by the Barclay Report (1982) when it advocated further delegation to front-line social workers.

Monitoring The assessment task identifies client needs at one point in time, but such needs may well change over time. In cases of chronic disability, there may be a gradually increasing need for extra services, followed by a point at which institutional care becomes necessary. In cases of acute illness, there is likely to be significant reduction in need after discharge and convalescence. So providing for changes in client need represents one rationale for the development of a monitoring system. Second, monitoring exercises enable practitioners to undertake self-evaluation of their work, within a task-centred framework, by specifying initial problems, identifying achievable goals and measuring the impact of intervention. This was a major objective of the case review system in both generic (Goldberg and Warburton, 1979) and elderly-specific forms (Crosbie, 1983). Thirdly, monitoring may also inform service providers about the effects different care packages have on client outcome. This is particularly important when innovatory activity is to be monitored, when the link between service and outcome may be almost unknown. Monitoring exercises can thus increase output mix efficiency by alerting workers to increases in need and augment input mix efficiency by signalling reductions in need.

What are the signs to look for in a high quality monitoring system? Such systems will cover a broad range of services (in some areas separate services may all be running their own partial monitoring systems), display formal report-back procedures, be based on continuous processes with set time limits, search for evidence from workers and informal helpers as well as from the client, and incorporate procedures for dealing with inadequacies in the light of such feedback.

Monitoring should produce continuous, descriptive information, and will usually be undertaken by the front-line workers who have allocated the services. In some cases more elaborate arrangements for audit or review of service provision are made, either by line managers or by a multidisciplinary panel where there is independence of the reviewers or the auditors from the original allocation decisions, providing opportunity for budgetary as well as professional review. In some assessment or rehabilitation units, periodic case conferences will be built into the case management process. Such reviews may also take place at the point of discharge from residential or hospital care.

Key worker Continuing service differentiation increases the premium placed on interservice co-ordination as a means of increasing market and input mix efficiency. The key worker system invests responsibility for such multiservice co-ordination in the hands of one designated worker. Such key workers have emerged in other areas, such as the care of the mentally handicapped (M. Plank, 1982), which require a multidisciplinary approach. Schemes may vary in their definition of the role of key workers. Such personnel will be especially valuable in systems which operate on a case conference basis, where key workers may prepare papers for consideration and have responsibility for the implementation of the care plan agreed. Often less well specified functions of co-ordination, securing resources and implementing monitoring systems will form the core of key workers' tasks.

Up to this point case management has represented the major theme in the improvement of service efficiency. But the enhancement of the content of the individual services being packaged is also of great importance in terms of output mix efficiency.

Direct work Counselling with elderly people has often been neglected (Rowlings, 1981) due to the perception of the elderly as a client group unlikely to experience positive change. Rowlings (1981) outlines ways in which direct work could be developed to handle issues of bereavement, loss, isolation and mental impairment which may be particularly prominent with elderly clients. An exploration of family psychodynamics may be crucial in making sense of a sudden request by carers for admission to residential or hospital care. These are output mix efficiency arguments.

But there is also a technical efficiency argument for direct work. Another technique includes matching procedures for client and helper, as is usually found with foster care placements for children, which are meant to reduce the risk of service breakdown. Such matching exercises can be found in many boarding out schemes (Ferlie, 1982) in which the social worker not only matches on the basis of interest but also provides ongoing support services. Matching is also seen as important in some voluntary schemes as a means of promoting a good volunteer/client relationship. Such matching is often on the basis of shared interests, but if volunteers take on 'heavier' tasks, attitudes towards incontinence, dementia, aggression and degree of acceptable risk could all be seen as important variables in a more complex matching process. Carers themselves may also provide self-help and counselling through relative support groups, which may or may not include social worker support.

Service variety and flexibility In analysing the extent of market and technical efficiency, *service variety* (differential responses in the light of different needs) and *service flexibility* (in time or in roles) form benchmarks by which services can be judged. Service content may well represent a more common focus for innovation than case management given the incremental nature of many innovations and the difficulties experienced in communicating laterally.

Enhanced service variety and flexibility is an important theme in a number of key services. The first example is the home help service. Although domestic care remains the backbone of the service (Howell, Boldy and Smith, 1979), it has moved towards the provision of out-of-hours, personal and specialist care. This increased service variety and flexibility augments the service's ability to respond to a wider range of needs. Such care will often respond to 'short interval needs' (Isaacs and Neville, 1976) as a means of re-establishing a daily support network, especially in the management of the demented.

The development of the nursing service as a means of coping with the needs of elderly people is a second area where changes in roles can be observed. The *Priorities* document (DHSS, 1976a) suggested a 6 per cent annual increase in nursing resources in order to enable the nursing service to support more elderly people in the community. Expansion may also pave the way for significant changes in roles and service quality. In hospital care continuing emphasis has been placed on the recruitment of more trained nurses following serious concern about the quality of nursing, especially in psychogeriatric settings. Here Arie and Jolley (1982) argue that in acute psychogeriatric wards the number of trained staff should at least equal untrained staff. In the community sector a process of role differentiation is apparent. The DHSS (1978) suggested the recruitment of more nursing auxiliaries to undertake personal care tasks for elderly people, with some overlap with the home help service. Additionally there are the new roles of community nurses and community psychiatric nurses attached to a hospital consultant but working in the community with greater case responsibility.

The third example of a service which stresses improvements in service content is very sheltered housing. Whereas conventional schemes relied on primitive forms of alarm systems and partial warden cover, very sheltered housing schemes often incorporate voice-to-voice mode alarms and total warden cover, based on higher staffing levels, relief wardens or a central call-in service (Ferlie, 1982). Very sheltered housing schemes pay attention to better physical design (Warwickshire SSD, 1980) and location to facilitate mobility. They typically make provision for extra home help and nursing support facilities so that admission to residential care can be avoided. However, wardens will often continue in their 'lay' role as attractors but not case managers of resources. So this service represents a good example of an area where improvements in service content outstrip enhancements in case management.

Short-term services Conventional service provision results in a split between a small 'in group' who receive long-term institutional care and a large 'out group' who rely on inadequate levels of very basic domiciliary services. The results of this mismatch of needs and resources have been demonstrated in areas such as sheltered housing (Heumann and Boldy, 1982) where, disability for disability, tenants receive 'overprovision' as wardens act as service magnets. There may also be a law of diminishing returns in at least some social services. Reid and Shyne's study (1969) of social casework found gains to be concentrated in more goal-directed and short-term casework. This points to the importance of developing short-term services in order to reduce silt-up and provide welfare gains for a larger number of clients. Such schemes may promote technical efficiency by maximising the benefits obtained from a given resource.

Short-term schemes include special post-discharge schemes to provide help over the critical resettlement period, relief care to support informal carers, and acute/assessment beds to provide an explicitly designed short-term service based on plans for early discharge. Arrangements for post-hospital discharge care represent a clearer focus for development than post-Part III care. Crisis intervention remains another way of providing short-term help, as the restoration of an equilibrium within a stressed family can obviate the need for admission to residential care. In the field of post-discharge care, Age Concern (1980) outlines the contribution that voluntary schemes can make to ease the transition from hospital to community care. The adoption of more flexible policies by residential care establishments marks an important area of development. Allen (1982) documents the recent rapid growth of short-stay admissions in Part III, concluding that the most common reasons for short-stay admission are to give either informal carer or the elderly client relief or a holiday. However, such increased client throughput also increases the workload for residential care staff.

Rehabilitation Some residents in long-term institutional care — estimates of those in residential care classified as of low dependency have been as high as 40 per cent (Booth, Barritt, Berry, Martin, Melotte and Phillips, 1982) — may not need full residential support if enhanced community services are available. Although other elderly people in the community may require such residential care, discharging the non-dependent elderly and admitting the more dependent will lead to a better matching of needs and resources. Because of the institutionalising effect of some residential care regimes on both physical and social independence, such discharges may be difficult to achieve. Rehabilitation thus contributes to technical efficiency by increasing the output of a given resource.

Many schemes attempt to improve functioning in a number of ways: physical rehabilitation through occupational therapy and physiotherapy; specific rehabilitative regimes for stroke, incontinence and depression; the promotion of coping strategies for clients exhibiting dementia and their relatives; and encouraging clients to increase their social skills and independence. Effective rehabilitation should at least in some cases arrest a drift into unnecessary long-term care.

Other signs

Some signs are not based directly on case-management or service content processes, although they have pervasive indirect consequences for the way in which these signs are handled.

Lower-cost mode Evidence relating to the cost hierarchy between care modes identified by the balance of care studies has already been examined in Chapter 1. The conclusion of the Audit Inspectorate study of services to elderly people was that there were pronounced cost differences between the three broad categories of care — hospital, residential or intensive domiciliary and less intensive domiciliary, and intensive domiciliary care was unlikely to be substantially more expensive than residential care to the public sector and will usually be cheaper to the local authority (Audit Inspectorate, 1983, p.22).

Tinker (1984) produces further evidence to show that community care innovations do indeed offer cost advantages to public agencies. Comparing the costs of innovatory schemes designed to care for elderly at home with other modes of provision, Tinker came to the following conclusion for elderly people of high dependency:

> As is known, hospital was by far the most expensive option and if the cost of land for any new building were included it would be even more so. The cost of a place in an acute hospital (£20,319) was more than three times the cost of Part III, sheltered housing or remaining at home with an innovatory scheme. In a geriatric or long-stay hospital it cost roughly double to care for an elderly person compared with elsewhere. For people who have no need to be there — and there are some — this is a very expensive option.

All the innovatory schemes (except the inner-city home care schemes and personal alarms) were cheaper than Part III and sheltered housing for people receiving a retirement or supplementary pension. They were still slightly cheaper than sheltered housing or Part III for people receiving every possible state income support including attendance allowance (Tinker, 1984, p.109).

The cost advantages of innovatory domiciliary-based schemes were even more apparent for elderly people of medium dependency. The innovations analysed by Tinker were service content-based, but many may also include a case management component. Such forms of modal shift will increase input mix efficiency. They often provide for the greater use of volunteers, support for informal carers so that they do not relinquish caring roles and greater use of lower-cost staff (such as auxiliary nurses) for tending tasks as a form of input substitution.

Support for informal carers The role of the informal carer is a subject of great debate. Feminists argue that community care policies are gender-loaded and substitute unpaid informal female labour for badly-paid formal female labour by privatising public burdens (Finch and Groves, 1983). Finch argues for a return to residential care-based policies, as part of a communal 'socialist' response:

> On balance, it seems to me that the residential route is the only one which ultimately will offer us a way out of the impasse of caring: collective solutions would, after all, be very much in the spirit of a socialist policy programme, and a recognition that caring is labour, and in a wage-earning economy should be paid as such, in principle should overcome some of the more offensive features of the various 'community' solutions (Finch, 1984, p.16).

The precise nature of the 'residential route' is neither elaborated nor costed. Nor is account taken of evidence in the care of other client groups (Bayley, 1973) that informal carers are likely to gain greater insight into individual needs of clients. Nor does this perspective pay sufficient attention to the preferences of elderly consumers or the mixed motives of many carers based on complex feelings of love, duty and guilt. The study by Levin, Sinclair and Gorbach (1982) of the supporters of demented elderly people, many of whom were carrying extremely heavy burdens, concluded:

> Their wish to care grew out of a pattern of life which was long-established and reinforced by bonds of affection and obligation. Forty-one per cent of the supporters were wives or husbands of the elderly clients and 44 per cent were their daughters or sons. Where the elderly clients and the supporters lived together this arrangement had been established on average for 36 years, and only 16 per cent of them had lived together for less than ten years.

> Most supporters said that they still felt close to their elderly relatives, that they still got satisfaction from helping them and that they still had good times together. The great majority wanted to keep their relatives at home. On initial interview, only 13 per cent of supporters indicated that they would definitely accept permanent care for their relatives in homes or hospitals if it was offered (ibid, p.234).

Informal care is well placed to respond to the unpredictable 'critical interval needs' (Isaacs and Neville, 1976) which require constant vigilance. However, the stress placed on many informal carers (Isaacs, Livingstone and Neville, 1972; EOC, 1982) has led to the argument that public agencies would be wise on grounds of efficiency as well as equity to invest in substantial support for those carrying out onerous duties in order to sustain them in their caring roles. The argument is that carer support is input mix efficient from the point of view of the public agency in the sustaining of informal inputs. Thus Neill's study (1981) of Part III admission procedures found that informal carers rarely received domiciliary services which could have prevented the strain reaching impossible levels. However, efficiency considerations dictate that resources should be allocated to those most likely to find their informal caring role unmanageable. In the care of elderly people the conditions which are least well tolerated by informal carers are dementia (Isaacs, Livingstone and Neville, 1972) and incontinence of faeces (Sanford, 1975). Priority status might also be accorded to those carers offering the greatest number of hours of care. Nissel and Bonnerjea (1982) estimate that over half the informal carers of dependent elderly people spend over three hours a day on caring on a long-term basis. The Equal Opportunities Commission (1982) found 44 per cent of informal carers had been caring for more than five years. Where there is no kin, neighbours and friends may be willing to help on a limited basis, but may soon relinquish their caring roles if statutory support is not forthcoming.

One efficiency argument against the provision of support for informal carers has been that formal and informal care act as substitutes rather than as complements. As public care is provided, so informal carers relinquish their role. There is now some preliminary evidence available (Frankfather, Smith and Caro, 1981) that such substitution effects are slight, except in those cases where public services are attempting to scale down the involvement of relatives to manageable levels. Yet Abrams (1977) has also argued that friends and neighbours, in particular where there is less of a kinship bond, might relinquish caring roles once statutory agencies have become involved. Although provisionally carer support can be justified on grounds of efficiency as well as equity, much more evidence is needed about substitution effects.

Production functions Even within a given service mode, there are a variety of organisational forms which will enhance or reduce technical efficiency (Williams and Anderson, 1975). One example is the adoption either of localised or centralised production systems according to whether large-scale production results in economies or diseconomies of scale for the function under consideration. The meals-on-wheels service is a good example of an area in which such technical questions assume significance.

Efficiency in the production process might also be expected to increase with the level of staff skill and management support which together constitute an important part of the stock of human capital. A serious criticism often made of services such as the home help service is that they are undermanaged with little co-ordination or planning capacity and with excessive lateral spans of control. The appointment of assistant home help organisers to carry out delegated tasks could indicate a strengthening of managerial capacity.

The use of low-cost or adapted resources is also indicative of a concern for non-capital intensive forms of development. Thus Babbage (1981) argues against the drift to capital intensive, very sheltered housing policies on the Warwickshire model on the basis that community-based alarm systems combined with an improvised day care facility could provide many of the benefits of conventional sheltered housing without the capital costs. In hospital settings, given stock can be redeployed to provide greater variety in the types of bed offered.

Sources of finance In a time of retrenchment, the importance of external sources of finance in the stimulation of innovation is well known (Glennerster et al., 1982). The provision of joint finance might affect the service content offered and the nature of case management processes. Indeed this will be the theme of a later chapter. At this point, the argument is solely that the provision of joint finance or other sources of external finance is likely to lead to better interagency co-ordination and allocation of resources, as individual agencies are forced to make at least minimal adjustment to the goals of other organisations and hence contribute to input mix efficiency.

Organisational Process

The argument has so far centred on the construction of an efficiency-based framework of signs which can be used to classify a mass of discrete product innovations. The *process* of change is a topic which should now be considered in addition to the *content* of change. The two may of course be linked as particular problem contexts or patterns of initiation may result in differential efficiency gains. There is a quantitative dimension to the process of innovation, as innovations may remain marginal 'showcase' programmes or be successfully replicated and thus exert significant changes in mainstream services. Many of the innovations reported were deeply embedded in the complexities of organisational life, requiring the negotiation of formal clearance and informal co-operation across a number of occupational groupings as well as the securing of finance in a cold economic climate. Market-based forms of innovation were not an issue; the central question revolved around the processes of organisational change. Professionally as well as managerially sponsored innovation (such as the formation of multidisciplinary teams) requires lateral negotiation across organisational boundaries, and possibly vertical clearance.

The information gathered on the organisational process of innovation in a postal trawl is of course more limited than that generated by an intensive processual case study of change and continuity in a single organisation (Pettigrew, 1985). Nevertheless it is important to go beyond the most simplistic rational and linear forms of innovation theory (evaluation leading to initiation leading to implementation leading to routinisation) to consider a wider range of process issues. A simplifying factor is that the level of analysis is predominantly at the level of discrete operational change rather than strategic change.

The overall framework adopted can be stated as follows. There are two key determinants in the adoption of an innovation. First, the calculation of the expected costs and benefits, economic and political, of innovating and not innovating. The decision makers making this calculation can be defined as the dominant coalition within the organisation or relevant suborganisation. Such dominant coalitions may change their nature over time. The second consideration is the capacity of the organisation to manage an accelerating rate of change. Each can be considered in turn.

Pressures towards stability and change

Following Hasenfeld (1983), the following can be seen as important sources of stability in human services organisations:

(i)   The need to preserve a location in a network and to have stable and predictable relations with key external agencies and professionals. Attempts to renegotiate boundaries between the SSD and the NHS may open a Pandora's box of issues which damage rather than enhance relations.

(ii) Innovation entails monetary and organisational costs to the adopting organisation as well as greater technological indeterminacy. All these costs are greatest to the earliest adopters (inventors rather than diffusors). SSDs used the rapid growth rates characteristic of the early 1970s for quantitative expansion rather than qualitative change. With the erosion of financial slack, SSDs find distress-based innovation difficult as funds have to be found from elsewhere in a pressurised budget. The incentive is to adopt alternative demand dampening devices such as waiting lists or cost shunting onto other agencies.

(iii) Organisational ideologies structure service intervention, providing a cognitive framework within which practititioners can operate. Changes in service systems therefore require legitimating ideologies.

(iv) There is a delicate internal power balance within many human service organisations which may be threatened by the process of innovation. In particular, dominant coalitions, while anxious to impose their own conceptions of strategic change, may resist definitions of the change process which threaten their dominance.

But there are also powerful pressures operating in favour of change:

(i) The continuing growth in the numbers of the very elderly, although the numbers of elderly are now beginning to decline. But it is the very elderly who make most intensive demands on services and who display a 'syndrome' of multiple needs, with social, medical and psychiatric components, who require multidisciplinary intervention. The demographic push is, however, locally variable: some areas (such as parts of Inner London) now have an elderly population which is significantly declining in size.

(ii) Changing patterns of funding. The historic downturn in the growth rate of SSD base budgets from the mid-1970s onwards and the increasing importance of external funding mechanisms such as joint finance designed to fulfill specific central objectives has important implications for service style. The rate of downturn in growth of course varies from one authority to another. The increased use of the social security budget as a funding mechanism for private residential care represents a form of cost shunting which may relieve the financial pressure facing the SSD.

(iii) Shifts in legislative and governmental policies. Such shifts may be less important in services for elderly people, where a minimalist pattern of central–local relations characterised the most recent statement of central policy (Cmnd 8173, 1981), than in services for mental health care groups, which have attracted much greater policy interest.

(iv) Changes in the policies and practices of key external agencies. Increased bed turnover in geriatric wards is a key policy issue in many health districts, often actively pursued by the new breed of acutely oriented geriatricians. The boundary between the nursing and home help service is becoming increasingly difficult to draw in some areas, as the nursing service responds to excess demand by attempting to hive off basic tending tasks to the home help service.

The organisational capacity to innovate

These contradictory pressures towards stability and change will be resolved differently from one area to another. But even where the pressures for change are dominant, the organisational capacity to respond to such changes varies according to:

Organisational structure Burns and Stalker's classic work (1961) suggested that in the private sector firms with an organic structure (role fluidity, a task rather than authority-centred structure, high levels of lateral communication) rather than a mechanistic structure (extensive role specialisation, a hierarchical system of control and high levels of vertical communication) display a higher degree of innovation. Human service organisations which are decentralised, low in formalisation and with highly diverse skills and knowledge might be thought to have a greater capacity to innovate (Hage, 1980). In more sophisticated versions different structures are seen as functional for particular types of innovation: incremental or radical, locally or centrally financed. These questions are explored further in Davies and Ferlie (1984) and Ferlie, Challis and Davies (1984).

Strategic choice Other writers have focused on the ability of organisational actors to define the task environment. Child (1972) argues that contingency theory failed to give due attention to the act of choice by the dominant coalition as decision makers were able to develop long-term organisational goals which in turn had implications for structure, technology and financial flows. Hage and Dewar's study (1973) of innovation in health and welfare agencies found that the commitment of executives towards change was the key predictor of the rate of programme innovation. Within human services organisations, the capacity of the centre to make and implement policy emerges as a crucial topic.

We were able to derive information on the following 'signs' of organisational process, which reflected some of the issues explored in the first part of the chapter.

Problem context Two main contexts can be outlined. The first is distress innovation: changes in service due to demographic growth, scarcity of Part III and hospital beds, or budgetary retrenchment which forces a closer examination of cost-effectiveness. Often such innovations will be based on technical efficiency arguments rather than allocative efficiency grounds and will display emphasis on such features as input substitution. The second context can be termed developmental innovation, certainly characteristic of the pre-1976 period of growth (Donnison et al., 1975) but perhaps also of those micro-climates protected from retrenchment today. Such innovations may often be launched by professionals who have internalised the aim of service development as an important facet of their work, partially as a legitimation of professional status. They may focus more on allocative efficiency considerations or indeed on non-efficiency based goals, concentrating on service development rather than optimal resource allocation.

Initiating personnel The various types of innovation can also be differentiated by their initiating personnel. There is a need to distinguish between *bottom-up*, *top-down* and *professional* perspectives which may result in very different innovatory processes.

Bottom-up innovations, designed to resolve specific bottlenecks and launched by front-line workers, may represent a characteristic mode of innovation in welfare agencies where initiative frequently passes to front-line workers (Lipsky, 1980). However, the weaknesses associated with such an approach may be considerable. Davies (1981b) argues that because personal social services innovations are often localised and incremental in nature, they are often weakly linked to the strategic issues facing agencies but respond to local perceptions of particular problems. The second danger is one of disjointed incrementalism: limited gains in one area may be achieved in isolation from similar changes in the rest of the service system. Single service enhancements of service content represent a good example of such processes. Third, bottom-up innovations may be unable to ensure the reallocation of significant departmental resources and may hence make only a limited impact in quantitative terms.

Professional innovations represent a second important source of organisational change. Both social workers and geriatricians have some scope to define legitimate changes in practice, but it is the latter who are subject to a much weaker form of state mediation in the producer/consumer relationship (Johnson, 1972) and who control significant resources. Indeed, the Ministry of Health directly encouraged the development of geriatric medicine as a new professional 'segment'. Such professionalised innovations may shift the pattern of service provision in a more systematic way than other front-line innovations. Changes in hospital admission and discharge policies will for example have major implications for SSDs.

Top-down innovation represents a third mode of change, usually defined as policies adopted at the centre of a SSD designed to be implemented at the periphery. These exercises will often be sponsored by senior management and can be related to strategic goals. Such approaches have been subject to criticism on the grounds that they fail to address issues of implementation, in particular lack of policy consensus and the complexity of implementing policies involving a multiplicity of actors. Some writers (Barrett and Fudge, 1981) have gone on from this to stress the role of discretion and local values as pervasive determinants of implementation processes. Yet it would be an error to underestimate the significant powers available to the centre of an SSD through, for example, earmarking resources for which local areas then have to compete on terms laid down by the centre. Second, on community care issues there may be both internal departmental consensus (although disagreement on how any new resources to finance community care programmes should be allocated between areas) and a limited number of occupational groupings. The implementation structure may be limited in scope. For example, an authority might decide to respond to increased demands produced by an ageing population by turning round the home help service into a home care service. This would be a strategic response involving changes in roles in response to long-term changes, but might not involve a variety of producer groups in implementation or even major issues of policy, given the extra status likely to accrue to the service in the event of re-organisation. Top-down innovation may play an important part in processes of organisational change.

Little is known about how these three modes of organisational change relate to efficiency gains. One hypothesis might be that non-professionalised front-line innovations aim at improved technical efficiency, whereas professionalised schemes aim at developmental rather than efficiency-based innovation but with some allocative efficiency gains in service content. Top-down innovations may be prompted by fiscal pressure but may sometimes move on to consider allocative efficiency both within the SSD and across agency boundaries where there is a major joint finance input.

Coverage Many innovations remain marginal to the overall pattern of service provision, and offer easier targets for expenditure reduction exercises than large established services (Davies and Ferlie, 1982). Attrition rates may be high or innovations may degenerate over time into pale imitations of their original conception. Innovatory roles may themselves become routinised, especially where they have been established by charismatic leaders who may eventually move to other posts or where there was an initial effect caused by a research presence.

In measuring the degree of scheme impact, the most evident indicators are first duration and second geographic spread. There is also the question of pilot status. The large number of innovations which take the form of pilot schemes, although certainly indicating efficiency is evaluated far more closely than in baseline practice, also indicates the vulnerability of many schemes in their reliance on short-term funding.

Joint working Central to the achievement of input mix and output mix efficiency is the recognition that care is provided by a service system, through resources which are substitutes and complements. Within such a system, care packaging in turn depends upon the achievement of interagency and interprofessional co-operation. Yet decision makers may continue to think in compartmentalised, departmentally-based terms (Glennerster, Korman and Marslen-Wilson, 1983). Greater co-ordination may be internal to an agency (between social workers and home help organisers), between agencies (social workers and nurses), and between public agencies and voluntary, neighbourhood and informal care. Indeed, one form of joint working consists of community development aimed at the generation of new forms of locally-based care.

Evaluation Evaluation is the precondition for the examination of the real world relationship between input and outcome as opposed to that hypothesised in the scheme protocol. Such evaluations should ideally measure final outcomes although many will concentrate on process criteria. Many innovations do not make any arrangement for evaluation and in those that do the task is carried out at various levels of sophistication ranging from progress reports by implementors to research designs involving in-house or external researchers.

Summary

The argument of this chapter can be summarised as follows. Innovation has been too often treated as a good in itself, rather than as a means of improving service efficiency. Although considerations of efficiency should ideally be measured on the basis of direct evidence about inputs and outcomes, there is also a tradition of process evaluation available based on definitions of 'good practice' which are associated with desired outcomes. The American quality assurance literature represents a useful starting point. A number of process criteria have been derived and provide a framework for the assessment of reported innovations in the care of elderly people. The argument that gains in efficiency might be linked to particular organisational settings was also introduced.

3 Innovation in the Home Help Service

Commentary

We now move from considering the development of a process-based framework for analysing the signs of efficiency improvement to the application of this framework to particular sectors of care. In this chapter we consider innovation in the home help sector. Five other sectors are considered in subsequent chapters.

The overall approach outlined in Chapter 2 was used to develop the coding framework for home help schemes. In order to compare the extent of efficiency improvement across the six care sectors identified, differences between the propensity of one care sector and the rest of the sectors to report the process-based signs of efficiency improvement were examined using chi-square tests. Only signs with at least five predicted positive observations could be included in the analysis in order not to violate statistical assumptions. Twenty-two such signs were identified for inclusion.

This chapter examines the characteristic features of home help innovation, using the 38 schemes reported in Ferlie (1982) as data. Key process signs are discussed in turn. In the second part of the chapter, two case studies are used to illustrate general arguments.

Domiciliary care is often thinly spread (D. Plank, 1977) with the result that intervention is not always concentrated on those individuals where welfare gains could be most sharply achieved. Associated with this have been poor allocation procedures both between individuals and between areas. Clients in one area might receive many more hours of home help time than clients in neighbouring areas, even though their dependency levels seemed similar. Some studies (Hurley and Wolstenholme, 1980) have found home helps performing tasks clients were able to do for themselves. The excessive span of control exercised by home help organisers (an average of 342 clients in 1979–80) has resulted in a relative neglect of assessment. The increase in 'thin spreading' can be seen in the fall of the estimated average number of hours per case from 4.7 in 1967 to 2.09 in 1979/80 (Hedley and Norman, 1982). So improved targeting would be expected to represent a major focus of efficiency improvement.

One way in which vertical target efficiency can be improved is through the introduction of eligibility criteria restricting access to those deemed to be in greatest need. Not only do some 75 per cent of home help innovations report the introduction of eligibility criteria, but this was found to be a significantly higher percentage than in the rest of the sample (Table 3.1). Home help schemes specified that clients should be frail or near the margin of admission to residential care (25 schemes), post-discharge cases (thirteen schemes) or lack sufficient informal carers (ten schemes).

The pursuit of greater vertical target efficiency should also reflect the fact that subgroups display characteristically different patterns of needs. For example, a home help service aimed at maintaining dementing elderly people in the community is likely to call for intensive out-of-hours care in order to be effective. However, Table 3.1 demonstrates that the home help service was less likely than the rest of the sample to report targeting on the basis of client subgroup. The client subgroups most likely to be targeted comprised elderly mentally infirm people (five schemes) and elderly physically handicapped people (four schemes). Thus although there is evidence of a substantial move to the greater targeting of innovatory home help resources, such targeting will often depend on a global measure of 'frailty' and rest on bureaucratically defined groups of cases such as those in post-discharge schemes and may neglect the development of a more varied service system able to care for distinct client subgroups.

Table 3.1
Signs of efficiency improvement:
home help sector compared
with other sectors

Sign		Chi square	Direction
1.	Targeting (eligibility criteria)	13.19***	positive
2.	Targeting (client subgroups)	8.64***	negative
3.	Uptake	5.72**	positive
4.	Outreach	4.84**	negative
5.	Assessment (enhanced type)	0.43	positive
6.	Assessment (multidisciplinary)	0.06	negative
7.	Care packaging	8.75***	positive
8.	Service arranging	0.43	positive
9.	Direct work	11.94***	negative
10.	Monitoring/follow-up	1 07	negative
11.	Key worker	1.37	positive
12.	Personal care	13.66***	positive
13.	Night sitting	11.85***	positive
14.	Out-of-hours working	14.48***	positive
15.	Short-term working	12.56***	positive
16.	Rehabilitation	0.54	negative
17.	Shift from institutional care	2.48	positive
18.	Support for informal carers	1.22	positive
19.	More efficient production process	2.74*	negative
20.	Joint finance	7.04***	positive
21.	Replication	2.34	positive
22.	Joint working with NHS	0.10	negative

Notes
* p at .10
** p at .05
*** p at .01
Source: Ferlie et al. (1984).

Horizontal target efficiency

The lack of horizontal target efficiency is also a matter of concern: indeed Bebbington and Davies (1983) argue that the home help service is characterised by a greater degree of horizontal than vertical target inefficiency. It is difficult to increase horizontal target efficiency if lack of uptake is based on an elderly person's reluctance to come to terms with increasing dependence or budgetary constraints on the volume of service available.

In other cases, a trade-off can be made between vertical and horizontal target efficiency. Certain service models emphasise the role of the home help or equivalent staff (such as patch workers) in securing early intervention on the basis of greater knowledge of client need (Cooper, 1980), particularly for elderly clients who may deteriorate rapidly in the absence of intervention. Such patch-based models stress accessibility and acceptability as a precondition for successful intervention. The advocates of a greater emphasis on horizontal target efficiency point to the need for an 'open' referral policy, the danger of assuming relative support which may not exist and the possible deterrent effect of charging. Hyman's (1981) study of the introduction of flat-rate charges for the home help service in Redbridge found that 366 clients (about 10 per cent) cancelled the service. Although many of these clients were the 'least' needy, there was also evidence that some high need clients cancelled.

Home help innovations were found to be significantly more likely than the rest of the sample to improve uptake (Table 3.1). Many post-discharge schemes do not impose charges, although the mainstream service may do so. An 'extensive' orientation is also observable in projects such as the Coventry Home Help Project which was originally set up to evaluate the effect of expansion of hours in one area, although an unanticipated pattern of qualitative differentiation also emerged.

This was offset by the finding (Table 3.1) that the sector was less likely than the rest of the sample to be undertaking outreach activity as a means of discovering new clients, unlike (say) welfare benefits campaigns. Indeed only one home help innovation reported outreach activity towards elderly mentally infirm people, despite the potential role of the service in maintaining elderly confused people at home and offering relief care to relatives (Hedley and Norman, 1982, p.33). Such specialist schemes already impose greater demands on staff in terms of unsocial hours worked and training needed and depend on complex organisational decision-making processes for implementation.

The home help sector also performed poorly on other measures of horizontal target efficiency. Home help innovations were in only three cases linked to preventive surveillance or screening exercises which could have increased the effectiveness of early intervention.

Case management

The mismatch between needs and resources is accentuated by poor provision both for initial assessment and for periodic reassessments. The management of a more flexible and varied service system which is responsive to changing levels of need calls for considerably more attention to be given to the assessment task. There is suspicion that

49

assessment may be based on moral judgements of 'deservingness' (Goldberg and Connelly, 1982, p.56) rather than the examination of a standard list of items and that reassessment is the first task to be abandoned when pressure of work becomes excessive. Home help innovations were not significantly more likely to report enhancements in the type of assessment (Table 3.1). Whereas Goldberg and Connelly (1982) argued that it would be beneficial to produce a 'check-list' to act as an aide-memoire for home help organisers, only three home help innovations reported the use of formal schedules. Four found less adventurous methods of improving assessment, such as greater attention to overall needs rather than assessing eligibility for one particular service.

However, as Goldberg and Connelly (1982, p.59) point out, if a common assessment form which covered a range of needs were to be devised, the problem would then emerge of who should administer the schedule: home help organiser, social work assistant or social worker. One of the reasons for the integration of the home help and fieldwork services within area teams was to improve communication between the two services. Thus the policy contained in DHSS Circular 53/71 (1971, p.4) stated that a referral for home help could lead to assessment for alternative kinds of assistance. Nevertheless Hedley and Norman (1982) found that in about 50 per cent of offices visited there was dissatisfaction with the relationship between social workers and home help organisers, sometimes involving complaints about abuse of service in cases involving possible Part III admission.

So efforts to move towards an agreed assessment of need take on crucial significance in home help innovations. Although there was almost exactly the same proportion of home help schemes as other schemes reporting some move to multidisciplinary assessment (Table 3.1), twelve home help innovations did report that social workers had become involved in the assessment process. In East Sussex's Hove Intensive Domiciliary Care Project, for example, a social worker was attached to the project partly to improve assessment skills. Such a displacement of home help organisers by social workers does not, however, correspond to the fullest definition of multidisciplinary assessment when the views of the social worker would be laid along-side those of a home help organiser who had been given the time and training to improve assessment skills.

Case management embraces a number of other techniques besides assessment. Of great interest in work with elderly people is care planning (Rowlings, 1981) or the pulling together of a number of traditionally isolated services into a coherent package. It has often been assumed that social workers rather than home help organisers would take on the role of care planner. However, in some schemes, home help organisers have taken on greater care planning tasks by increasing their span of control to allocate a range of domiciliary services and could be given enhanced executive power to arrange these services. One disadvantage of this approach is that links with area teams may remain weak. Additionally, such a home care organiser model assumes reductions in numbers of clients and workers carried by each organiser, together with improved supervision, support, and assessment and re-assessment procedures.

Table 3.1 indicates that home help schemes were significantly more likely than other schemes to report some form of care packaging. Although care packaging arrangements often remained rudimentary, six schemes explicitly reported that organisers were expected to tailor a range of services to meet individual need. For example the Kirklees Home Care Scheme is managed by a home care organiser who supervises her own team of staff and who has direct management responsibility for all domiciliary resources (home help, warden and meals-on-wheels) provided to the client. However, only eighteen out of the 38 home help schemes reported some form of care packaging, indicating continuing neglect of basic case management tasks even in innovative schemes. More effective care packaging may be associated with the form of central departmental organisation. Thus Harbert and Dexter (1983, p.58) quote London evidence which suggests that the move to integration of domiciliary services at local level is associated in turn with the existence of a centrally-based organiser at HQ.

One development has been termed the 'social service officer' role, similar to the Domiciliary Services Officers in Nottinghamshire or Social Services Officers in East Sussex (Hey, 1980). The term is defined as follows:

> The difference between this model and the extended home help organiser role lies not in any interaction of worker and client but in the fact that the new professional does not manage a team of 'helps' as does the home care organiser (Hey, 1980, pp.101-2).

These posts are one tier removed from front-line supervision and concentrate on assessment of client need across the basic services field and on arranging provision. These officers would be able to make a detailed request for deployment of particular kinds of home help. Only a very few schemes reported such posts, but they are of growing significance. Clearly any move in this direction would be welcome given the present picture of concentration on programming (Gwynne, 1980) rather than supervision, assessment and care planning.

After the initial care package has been set up, it should be adjusted to changes in needs. However, only seven schemes reported monitoring procedures which would have enabled organisers to adjust services to changing patterns of need. This is disappointing in view of the suspicion that services may be continued long after the need for them has disappeared. Only six schemes made arrangements for internal audit and review of performance, with outside scrutiny of allocation decisions unheard of. Other case management features were also weakly represented within the home help section: one-quarter of home help innovations made arrangements for a key worker system, as opposed to one-half of those in the social worker/assessment/ rehabilitation category. Such key workers as were available concentrated on co-ordination roles rather than stronger ones such as implementing an agreed care plan.

Many case management tasks are neglected within home help innovations, despite incremental expansion of home help organiser roles to encompass other domiciliary services. There is also evidence that continued service differentiation has led to management fragmentation with the creation of additional line management hierarchies to manage new personal care services.

Service content

Not surprisingly, Table 3.1 indicates that home help innovations were less likely to report the provision of direct work than the rest of the sample. However, a central theme is the move towards the provision of a home care service. This was reported by three-quarters of the home help innovations and this sector was significantly more likely than the rest of the sample to report the provision of personal care (Table 3.1). But such a shift raises a number of key questions. What are the defining limits of the policy? Up to what degree of dependency can elderly clients be maintained in the community? How demanding is a pattern of unsocial working on staff? When will the nursing service begin to complain about duplication? Hammersmith and Fulham Home Carers are for instance expected to work a flexible week of 36 hours within a 24-hour, seven days a week service and to undertake washing and bathing tasks. The Berkshire Home Aides are expected to carry out tasks normally performed by different groups of health and social services staff.

The organisation of these home care services also raises important issues. An incremental move to more personal care within the mainstream service offers an alternative model of development to the creation of specialist squads. Reports gave too few details of specific tasks undertaken by home carers for detailed analysis but it would be most interesting to discover whether they undertake work relating to lifting, bed sores or medication. There is a danger that the move to personal care might be caught up in a desire to improve the status of the service and to achieve substitute nurse status (Harbert and Dexter, 1983, p.201) rather than a consideration of client needs. As Hedley and Norman (1982, p.34) argue, the organisational pluralism associated with the emergence of home care schemes may hide a lack of clear thinking concerning the roles, training or organisation implied by such a shift.

It seems that home help innovations are based on the enhancement of service content and display a relative neglect of case management. This is confirmed by the fact that night-sitting and out-of-hours services were significantly more frequent in this sector than the rest of the sample (Table 3.1). Thus twelve home help schemes reported a night-sitting service, as opposed to only two in the case management category. Again seventeen home help schemes reported an out-of-hours service as opposed to seven in the case management category. For a service which has sometimes been criticised as inflexible due to employment legislation and agreements as well as a work culture which emphasises mass programming rather than individual tailoring, this represents an important move towards greater service flexibility. A good example of this approach is Bradford's Night Care Service which provides a short-term intensive sitting-in service for 'at risk' client groups and also provides short-term intensive help to facilitate planned Part III admissions.

Cost-related criteria

One response to a shallow need/allocation gradient has been the provision of time-limited service to meet short-term needs. Such services often provide for the needs of elderly people who have been recently discharged from hospital where otherwise there might be a gap in arrangements for care or who are at risk of institutional admission for social reasons. Table 3.1 indicates that the move to short-term care, where the time commitment is usually automatically specified, is significantly greater in the domiciliary care sector than in the rest of the sample. The 26 home help innovations which report short-term working can be further broken down into subcategories: twelve reported crisis work, nine post-hospital discharge care and seven relief care for relatives. Although only fifteen schemes in the SSD support services sector (Chapter 5) reported short-term services, nine of these involved relief care. The home help service seems to place a lower priority on supporting relatives than other objectives such as freeing a hospital bed or preventing admission to Part III.

There are of course problems in delivering short-term services. Programming becomes even more complex and needs are often underestimated in post-discharge schemes so that organisers are faced with difficult choices. In order to avoid abandoning frail and needy clients, organisers will either have to negotiate handing over clients to the mainstream home help service, perhaps able to offer only a less intensive service, or continue with the 'short-term' scheme so that turnover drops and the NHS is less able to discharge patients. The Age Concern (Gateshead) post-discharge scheme reported just such a silting-up process (Ferlie, 1982).

As far as rehabilitation was concerned, the home help sector was almost exactly as likely as the rest of the sample to report such activity. Of the sixteen schemes reporting rehabilitative activity in this sector, most concentrated on physical rehabilitation, often linked to a post-hospital discharge scheme. Only one scheme reported work developing coping strategies for elderly mentally infirm people and their carers, which takes the debate back to the level of training which should be offered to specialist home helps.

The sector was significantly more likely to report a shift to lower cost modes of care (Table 3.1). In particular, 33 schemes reported an intention to shift care for marginal clients from institutional to community modes. Although the home help sector was more likely than the rest of the sample to provide support for informal carers, this relationship was not significant. Nevertheless the voluntary sector (Chapter 8) reported a much higher percentage of schemes aimed at supporting informal carers. Why the home help sector should perform relatively poorly on this item is an important question: perhaps as a mass programming service it finds difficulty in meeting the individual needs of informal carers. Perhaps sexist allocation policies persist so that the needs of female carers for support are not taken seriously. General Household Survey evidence suggests that the home help service is far more likely to be provided to married couples when it is the wife who is disabled (and hence the husband is the carer) than vice versa (Bebbington and Davies, 1983, p.319).

The sector was significantly less likely than the rest of the sample to report a move towards a more efficient production process (Table 3.1). Despite the argument that a move towards a more flexible, varied and responsive service requires substantial investment in improved training and management support, only seven schemes reported a concern with improving training and six with management support. The legacy of inadequate training and underresourced management threatens to blight attempts to provide a service aiming at a high level of home help and organiser skill. The Younghusband Report (1959) failed to give a clear impetus to home help organiser training with the result that organisers traditionally relied on a National Association of Local Government Officers (NALGO) correspondence course and then Certificate in Social Service (CSS) courses for their training needs. However, the CSS course has been designed for junior staff in the social work profession (such as social work assistants) rather than home help organisers moving into management roles. So home help organisers have been thrown back on to their own resources.

Ferlie (1982) provides examples of the type of training and management tasks now being undertaken, such as courses to train home helps to recognise the signs of dementia. In order to free the time of home help organisers for management rather than programming tasks, Warwickshire has provided additional support. The Coventry Home Help Project led to the fuller integration of the home help organiser as a member of the area team.

Finance

Domiciliary care schemes are normally financed either by SSD base budget money (21 schemes) or joint finance (nineteen schemes). Table 3.1 demonstrates that home help innovations are significantly more likely to be joint financed than the rest of the sample. The role of joint finance can be seen most obviously in post-discharge schemes. Whether these new patterns of service are replicated to cover other elderly clients or remain isolated segments remains to be seen. Although externally financed innovation remains extremely important in domiciliary innovations, over half the domiciliary care schemes include base budget money showing that internal processes are also at work. Given the strategic role of the domiciliary care sector, it is worrying that there should be so little attention to improving inter-service case management despite the presence of external funding.

Organisational process

The key problem context seems to be bed-blocking, as pressure on Part III beds (23 schemes) or hospital beds (ten schemes) formed the largest categories reported. Such 'bottlenecks' were more important than general budgetary pressure (only two schemes) or the perceived failure of existing services (ten schemes) in explaining why these innovations were launched. Thus the Bexley Home Care Pilot Scheme grew from the appointment of a new geriatrician with an acute discharge policy, with the result that long-term geriatric beds were decreasingly available. The concentration on relieving pressure on institutional care concords with the incremental, 'bottleneck solving', service content-based nature of many home help innovations.

Such innovatory processes might be thought of as 'bottom up' (Webb, 1978) in nature and as particular responses to local problems.

55

Information given on the initiating personnel behind each innovation did not, however, bear this out. Thus whereas home help organisers were reported to initiate two schemes, SSD central working parties were reported to lie behind seven schemes, and local NHS/SSD groups five others. Even 'top down' innovations often remain incremental in nature. Of course there are exceptions: Bradford SSD reports a strategic development programme in its home help service. Nevertheless the failure to effect more radical forms of development is noteworthy. Many home help innovations remained tender plants: eleven of the schemes had only achieved pilot status, and only three had effected a transition to post-pilot permanence. Only six schemes reported a life of more than five years. Marginality continues to plague many home help innovations (Davies and Ferlie, 1982) with the relationship between innovatory and mainstream services remaining problematic. Although domiciliary care sector schemes were rather more likely than the sample as a whole to extend coverage beyond one geographical area (Table 3.1), this difference was not significant.

Information was also recorded on the extent to which collaborative joint working was developed with other agencies and resources (Table 3.1). Domiciliary care innovations were almost exactly as likely as the sample as a whole to report joint working with the NHS: but this accounted only for fourteen of the 38 schemes. The service with which the closest links had been built up was undoubtedly the nursing service, with which eleven schemes reported joint working. In some cases the development of this liaison was a central feature of the innovation, as in the North Tees Home Care scheme in which home care and home nursing staff are based at the same centre and are seen as alternative resources used according to the level of dependency of the client. Better internal liaison was usually established with field-work services (twelve reports) rather than day care (three reports) or residential care services (two reports).

Discussion

A first theme relates to the role of the home help organiser. Comments on the lack of integration of services reflect dissatisfaction with present concentration on programming a large part-time workforce. Various approaches have been tried but the two main options appear to be either the appointment of specialist home care organisers responsible for smaller caseloads or the elevation of senior home help organisers into social services officer roles supported by extra clerical or junior organiser staff. The first establishes new personal care roles more forcefully in the specialist service (there may be a danger that innovations erode over time) whereas the latter approach facilitates the care packaging of basic services, with emphasis on personnel management and programming tasks.

A second issue relates to the development of personal care tasks. Hedley and Norman (1982) argue that the rapid move to such intensive care could be proceeding without clear definitions of the training needed, the tasks to be performed and job grading. Many job descriptions seem vague, referring only to the 'care expected of a relative'. The arrangements for employment of home carers also varies: one scheme deemed them to be self-employed, another paid them at the home help rate plus 15 per cent and a third paid them at nursing auxiliaries rates. It may be that the need for extra skills will emerge as the schemes develop over time. A few schemes already refer to the increasing need for home carers to have knowledge of work with elderly mentally infirm people. What are the defining limits of this policy? In particular, how closely do home carers move towards basic nursing? The renegotiation of roles in the domiciliary care sector will prove of major importance in shaping what is the basic care service for many elderly people.

Third, there seems to be an excessive concentration on incremental, service content-based innovations with a relative neglect of case management functions. The danger is that service differentiation will lead to service fragmentation with poor lateral communications across an increased number of services. In addition, some schemes have reported difficulties in the implementation of radical forms of innovation. For instance Surrey's Community Support Scheme for elderly people failed to achieve original 'care packaging' objectives and found it difficult to recruit home helps willing to work out of hours. Many domiciliary care innovations are still doing too little, too late.

Case Studies

The case studies which follow illustrate how the classification framework we developed can be applied and how differences emerge when apparently similar innovations are studied.

Coventry Social Services Department: Home Help Project

This scheme underwent a shift from originally limited concerns about increasing expenditure to complex changes in the pattern of service provision. That this shift happened in an informal and unplanned way demonstrates the possibility that even incremental schemes may sometimes result in considerable service enhancements.

The Coventry scheme did not originally set out to serve any

particular subgroups. Its aim was to double the amount of home help hours in one area of the city in order to examine the argument that there existed substantial amounts of unmet need within the community (see Table 3.2).

Unexpected developments in the role of the home help organiser in the direction of greater integration with the area team emerged. Her assessment of need was utilised in relation to other services, and she accepted their assessment of need for home help. Occasionally, a joint assessment with a social worker was made when casework involvement was indicated. The organiser also initiated and processed applications for other basic services and encouraged and assisted in claims for benefits. This emphasis on securing resources can be seen as creating new 'key worker' tasks for the organiser. Unlike the Kirklees or Bexley schemes, however, full-blown care planning mechanisms did not emerge.

Turning to the home helps themselves, the proportion of time spent on cleaning tasks fell considerably and time spent providing personal care rose, and some clients received late evening or early morning visits. In addition, workers gradually developed special expertise in caring for post-hospital discharge cases, stroke victims, the deaf or the demented. Service provision thus underwent a considerable degree of differentiation.

The scheme provided a short-term service through a mobile emergency home help who provided a free service for up to a month for people discharged from hospital or experiencing a crisis. An assessment exercise showed that many scheme clients were dependent enough for institutional care. In addition, the project also seemed to have reduced the need for scarce community nursing resources. Emphasis was also placed on improving the training and support of home helps. A more selective recruitment policy was introduced and the organiser given extra support. The authority was able to attract outside funds to support the project from trusts and the DHSS.

There is little information on how the scheme was initiated. It is clear, however, that it was initiated for developmental reasons: a dissatisfaction with the impact of existing services. The project was conceived in terms of a one-off pilot exercise which has now run its course. Although there has since been SSD-wide re-organisation, it would be interesting to discover to what extent unplanned gains were 'halo effects' associated with the innovatory phase which are difficult to replicate.

Weak relationships are apparent with the health service (compare this with the Bexley scheme), but wardens in sheltered housing were supervised directly by the home help organiser. Emphasis was also placed on developing links between the home help service and the rest

58

Table 3.2
Coventry SSD Home Help Project:
case finding

Dimension	Response
Targeting (eligibility criteria)	No/no mention
Targeting (client subgroups)	No/no mention
Uptake	Intention to raise uptake, e.g. introduction of free service. creation of more accessible resources
Outreach	No/no mention
Mandatory assessment	No/no mention
Preventive surveillance	No/no mention

Table 3.3
Coventry SSD Home Help Project:
case management

Dimension	Response
Assessment (type)	General commitment
Assessment (inputs)	Social workers Home help organisers
Care packaging (type)	No/no mention
Care packaging (scope)	No/no mention
Arranging for additional services	Negotiating procedure for arranging other services by the SSD and by other agencies
Direct work	General commitment
Monitoring (type)	No/no mention
Monitoring (scope)	No/no mention
Monitoring (by whom?)	No/no mention
Audit/review?	No/no details
Key worker (role)	Securing other SSD and non-SSD services
Key worker (who?)	Home help organisers
Post-institutional care review	Home help organisers

**Table 3.4
Coventry SSD Home Help Project:
care provision**

Dimension	Response
Personal care	General commitment
Domestic care	General commitment
Night sitting	No/no mention
Out-of-hours working	Yes
Specialist care (eligibility criteria)	Post-discharge care
Specialist care (client subgroups)	Elderly mentally infirm Stroke patients Deaf

**Table 3.5
Coventry SSD Home Help Project:
efficiency**

Dimension	Response
Short-term commitment	Post-discharge (hospital) Crisis work
Rehabilitation	No/no mention
Lower-cost mode	Shift from institutional care Use of lower-cost staff
Support for informal carers	No/no mention
More efficient production process	Training Improved management support
Source of finance	SSD base budget DHSS Private (trust)

of the area team. Finally, unlike the other case studies, a substantial evaluation was undertaken by a specially appointed research officer on the (limited) question of accounting costs to the agency.

Conclusion The Coventry scheme illustrates the complex knock-on effects which may materialise even in initially simple designs. This should not be exaggerated: case-finding techniques and relations with

Table 3.6
Coventry SSD Home Help Project:
organisational process

Dimension	Response
Problem context	Observed failure of present service
Initiating personnel	No/no mention
Pilot?	Pilot scheme - now terminated
Duration	Less than 5 years
Coverage	One district only

Table 3.7
Coventry SSD Home Help Project:
joint working

Dimension	Response
Joint working (NHS staff)	No/no details
Joint working (housing department staff)	Sheltered housing wardens
Individual volunteers	No/no details
Voluntary organisations	No/no details
New forms of internal cross working	Domiciliary care division Fieldwork service division
Evaluation (by implementors)	No/no details
Evaluation (by other internal officers)	SSD research and development section
Evaluation (by external evaluators)	No/no details

other agencies remained mainly unaltered. But while there were no full-scale shifts to care planning, there were certainly moves in that direction. Major developments also took place in the role of the home help organiser and service. The Coventry scheme thus steadily developed in a less incremental direction towards effecting major changes.

The Kirklees Home Care Scheme

One of the crucial themes in the development of domiciliary services is the relationship between differentiation and integration. Given increased specialisation, how is co-ordination to be achieved? The Kirklees Home Care Scheme offers one approach to this dilemma, combining the provision of a new home care service with concentrated organisational responsibility for delivery of all domiciliary resources.

Table 3.8 indicates that the main achievements did not lie in the case-finding field. Gains were achieved in terms of client uptake (by providing a seven-day-a-week and out-of-hours emergency service). It was also expected that the home care service would be available at short notice. These could represent major gains for clients. In addition the scheme is available to all clients who are deemed to require a daily intensive service for a short period of time so it is targeted on clients with a particular level of need or particular conditions. There are, however, no signs of outreaching into the community to provide new services for hard-to-reach clients, nor of encouraging new referrals by screening devices such as preventive surveillance.

Table 3.8
Kirklees SSD Home Care Scheme:
case finding

Dimension	Response
Targeting (eligibility criteria)	On margin of need for residential care/frail
Targeting (client subgroups)	No/no mention
Uptake	Intention to raise uptake, e.g. introduction of free service, creation of more accessible resources
Outreach	No/no mention
Mandatory assessment	No/no mention
Preventive surveillance	No/no mention

Table 3.9 indicates that the scheme does indeed emphasise enhanced case management features. The assessment arrangements specify that the service will only be provided on the basis of a full assessment and treatment plan, to be made by a social worker (preferably level 3) and the home care organiser. A second feature of the scheme is the emphasis on domiciliary care planning. The special home care service is provided through a home care organiser (directly responsible to the home help organiser) who also has direct management responsibility for other domiciliary services, namely wardens and meals-on-wheels, which can be arranged directly by the home care organiser. The service is also reviewed every seven days to ensure it is still necessary.

As far as the home care service is concerned, the greater changes took place in the night sitting and out-of-hours facilities rather than

Table 3.9
Kirklees SSD Home Care Scheme:
case management

Dimension	Response
Assessment (type)	General commitment
Assessment (inputs)	Social workers Home help organisers
Care packaging (type)	Tailoring
Care packaging (scope)	SSD domiciliary care Sheltered housing
Arranging for additional services	Negotiating procedure for arranging other services by the SSD
Direct work	No/no mention
Monitoring (type)	No/no mention
Monitoring (scope)	No/no mention
Monitoring (by whom?)	No/no mention
Audit/review?	General commitment
Key worker (role)	Implementing care plan
Key worker (who?)	Home help organisers
Post-institutional care review	No/no mention

the actual tasks performed (see Table 3.10). No mention was made of links with nursing services, nor of new personal care tasks but only of more intensive domestic care tasks. The care aides' grading and conditions are indeed identical to those of home helps, with extra payments for unusual hours. So changes in the actual tasks performed, although significant, have been of an incremental rather than whole-sale nature.

Table 3.11 indicates the ways in which the scheme can be judged to improve efficiency. A short-term service is the basis of the whole method of working, not only in the availability of crisis working but

Table 3.10
Kirklees SSD Home Care Scheme:
care provision

Dimension	Response
Personal care	No/no mention
Domestic care	General commitment
Night sitting	Yes
Out-of-hours working	Yes
Specialist care (eligibility criteria)	On margin of need for institutional care
Specialist care (client subgroups)	No/no mention

Table 3.11
Kirklees SSD Home Care Scheme:
efficiency

Dimension	Response
Short-term commitment	Crisis work
Rehabilitation	No/no mention
Lower-cost mode	Shift from institutional care
Support for informal carers	No/no mention
More efficient production process	Training
Source of finance	SSD base budget

Table 3.12
Kirklees SSD Home Care Scheme:
organisational process

Dimension	Response
Problem context	Observed failure of present service: excessive rigidity
Initiating personnel	No/no mention
Pilot?	No/no mention
Duration	Less than 5 years
Coverage	Several districts

also due to the requirement that the service be provided for limited periods (up to six weeks) and be subject to review every seven days. Although this may well prevent unnecessary admissions to residential care, there was little reported emphasis on rehabilitation programmes or support for relatives under stress, which might also have this effect. However, there is provision for training organisers and aides in performing their new tasks. The scheme is financed by the SSD base budget and there are no external subsidies.

Table 3.12 indicates that the scheme was seen in developmental terms: the need to reduce service rigidity. Although it is not a pilot scheme and is proceeding in at least two teams, its marginality is indicated by its very recent origin. Although the scheme does provide for a joint assessment with a social worker its links with other resources are weak, even with nursing services (see Table 3.13). Finally, the scheme is to be monitored by the SSD's research officer and principal assistant (domiciliary services). The Kirklees scheme is unusual in specifying so explicitly arrangements for assessment, review and care planning. To counterbalance these strengths there seems less awareness of the need to develop the tasks performed or to build links with related agencies. It is to this subject that the last scheme in this section returns.

Table 3.13
Kirklees SSD Home Care Scheme:
joint working

Dimension	Response
Joint working (NHS staff)	No/no details
Joint working (housing department staff)	No/no details
Individual volunteers	No/no details
Voluntary organisations	No/no details
New forms of internal cross working	Domiciliary care division Fieldwork service division
Evaluation (by implementors)	No/no details
Evaluation (by other internal officers)	SSD research and development section
Evaluation (by external evaluators)	No/no details

Bexley Social Services Department: Home Care Pilot Scheme

The Bexley Home Care Pilot Scheme is noteworthy as one of the very few innovations which combines care packaging with the involvement of the NHS. Services available to be tailored included home

Table 3.14
Bexley SSD Home Care Pilot Scheme:
case finding

Dimension	Response
Targeting (eligibility criteria)	On margin of need for residential care/frail Post-discharge care
Targeting (client subgroups)	No/no mention
Uptake	No such intention/mention
Outreach	General commitment
Mandatory assessment	No/no mention
Preventive surveillance	No/no mention

help, social work and district nursing. The project also had access to the local geriatric unit and geriatrician, occupational therapist and day hospital.

As Table 3.14 indicates, the project was aimed at helping elderly people (up to a maximum of ten) who would otherwise require Part

Table 3.15
Bexley SSD Home Care Pilot Scheme:
case management

Dimension	Response
Assessment (type)	Focus on problem/strengths rather than eligibility for service Formal instrumentation used: schedule for physical capacity Assessment at home and in day unit
Assessment (inputs)	Social workers OTs/physiotherapists Geriatricians
Care packaging (type)	Tailoring Emphasis on supporting/increasing inputs from informal carers
Care packaging (scope)	SSD domiciliary care SSD fieldwork services NHS community services Day hospitals Voluntary inputs
Arranging for additional services	Negotiating procedure for arranging other services by the SSD and by other agencies
Direct work	General commitment
Monitoring (type)	No/no mention
Monitoring (scope)	No/no mention
Monitoring (by whom?)	No/no mention
Audit/review?	No/no details
Key worker (role)	Prepares papers for case conferences
Key worker (who?)	Social workers
Post-institutional care review	No/no mention

III or hospital care — including those who refused to leave their own home even if offered alternative residential care — and enabling clients to remain in the community or be discharged from inappropriate hospitalisation back into the community and enhancing their quality of life. There is outreach to frail elderly people at home unwilling to accept residential care, but this relates only to a small number of clients and more extensive methods of improving uptake are not used.

Major emphasis is placed on assessment and care planning. As Table 3.15 indicates, client applications are accompanied by a client profile form. This gives a detailed description of accommodation, client's ability and help available from other sources. This is considered at working party meetings with the help of the geriatrician

Table 3.16
Bexley SSD Home Care Pilot Scheme:
care provision

Dimension	Response
Personal care	Bathing/washing
Domestic care	Shopping
	Preparation of meals
Night sitting	Yes
Out-of-hours working	Yes
Specialist care (eligibility criteria)	On margin of need for institutional care
	Post-discharge care
Specialist care (client subgroups)	Incontinent

and occupational therapist. The tailoring exercise builds in volunteer help where this is available in particular cases. Social work support is available along with home help (up to 21 hours per week, usually split into two or more visits per day) as is district nursing for early morning and twilight work. Day hospital attendance for bathing and assessment has been included in some plans. The social worker is expected to act not only as co-ordinator and assessor but also to undertake direct work with clients by being aware of the emotional needs of clients who face increasing disability, to help maintain or increase the quality of their lives. Although the social workers play a key role in preparing case conference papers, other aspects of case management, such as periodic monitoring of services offered, remain at an informal level.

The scheme offers a range of support. Domestic but not personal care is provided by the home help service and meals-on-wheels service, and personal care by the day hospital (for bathing), and nursing care is provided by the district nursing service, including an out-of-hours service. As Table 3.16 shows, one of the unplanned developments in the scheme was the necessity to cope with incontinence: a serious problem in more than half the caseload. An incontinence laundry service would greatly assist the scheme. The scheme thus manages to offer a variety of services, at various levels of need.

The scheme is not just a short-term post-discharge scheme but also works towards longer-term alternatives to institutional care. As Table

Table 3.17
Bexley SSD Home Care Pilot Scheme: efficiency

Dimension	Response
Short-term commitment	No/no mention
Rehabilitation	Physical rehabilitation
Lower-cost mode	Shift from institutional care Support for informal carers Use of volunteers
Support for informal carers	Domiciliary care Volunteers
More efficient production process	Training
Source of finance	SSD base budget NHS base budget

3.17 also shows, the medical inputs mean that physical rehabilitation is available.

Relations with the geriatrics unit are excellent, so phased discharges and emergency short-term readmissions are possible. The scheme aims at reducing the need for long-term care, supporting informal carers and using volunteers (all of which have cost consequences) but also goes on to develop staff skills. Home helps often discuss their cases with members of the geriatric unit in order to learn how best to work with their clients. The funding for this pilot project came from NHS and SSD base budgets, and joint finance was not involved.

The scheme was sparked off by general worries about the increased pressure on hospital and Part III places, expressed through a local working party which combined SSD and NHS personnel (Table 3.18). It is a pilot scheme operating in one division, and so as yet of marginal significance, although a similar scheme is also planned for the central division.

Although relationships between NHS and SSD personnel were close, links with the housing department were not mentioned. Although volunteers were used, plans to use paid volunteers could not be implemented after discussions with the borough legal department.

Table 3.18
Bexley SSD Home Care Pilot Scheme:
organisational process

Dimension	Response
Problem context	Observed failure of present service: disregard of client preferences
	Pressure on OPH beds
	Pressure on hospital beds
	Demographic trends
	Budgetary pressures
Initiating personnel	Joint working: local NHS/SSD group
Pilot?	Yes
Duration	Less than 5 years
Coverage	One district only

Table 3.19
Bexley SSD Home Care Pilot Scheme:
joint working

Dimension	Response
Joint working (NHS staff)	Nurses/nursing officers
	Geriatricians
	Day care staff
	OTs
Joint working (housing department staff)	No/no details
Individual volunteers	Yes
Voluntary organisations	No/no details
New forms of internal cross working	Domiciliary care division
	Fieldwork service division
Evaluation (by implementors)	Yes
Evaluation (by other internal officers)	No/no details
Evaluation (by external evaluators)	No/no details

4 Innovation in the Case Management Sector

Commentary

The second group of schemes consists of 26 innovations (Ferlie, 1982), including not only social work activity but also assessment and rehabilitation-based schemes. Although the smallest of the three SSD sectors in terms of numbers, it is important as the sector most likely to enhance case management rather than service content tasks. Coded-up information and detailed examples are again taken from Ferlie (1982) and Ferlie, Challis and Davies (1983). These reports should be studied in relation to a literature which is now critical of the secondary status accorded to social work with elderly people (Goldberg and Warburton, 1979; Rowlings, 1981). Thus Holme and Maizels (1978) demonstrate that the more junior the grade of social worker, the more likely that worker was to carry elderly cases and the less likely to carry child care cases. Junior workers also carried larger caseloads, which limited the application of case management skills. Studies in urban (Goldberg and Warburton, 1979) and rural (Grant, 1981a,b) settings show that the majority of elderly clients are assessed, receive some information, and are then put in touch with practical services. In addition there is also a substantial elderly chronic population who receive occasional review visits. Goldberg and Warburton (1979) estimated that only about 10 per cent of elderly referrals, mainly very frail or confused, received more active and intensive social work support over an extended period.

Goldberg and Warburton (1979, p.128) distinguish between elderly people who can manage on their own with the help of domiciliary or other practical services, those who need to be in close touch with a supportive helping network and those who also require skilled social work help. The failure to maintain these distinctions means that planning for long-term care may become unnecessarily haphazard in nature. Many of those on the margin of Part III admission would benefit from case management skills. For example, admission to institutional care could be precipitated by the death of a relative which destroys the existing network of informal care or a refusal by the family to continue caring, unless practical and emotional support is made available.

So case management-based schemes might be expected to emphasise vertical target efficiency. In fact, while they were more likely to report targeting arrangements by eligibility criteria than the rest of the sample, the difference was not significant (Table 4.1). Such targeting arrangements that did exist within the sector were concentrated on two particular groups: elderly people at the margin of admission to residential care, and post-discharge schemes. The construction of a comprehensive support network is particularly emphasised in the management of dementing elderly at home. However, case management schemes were rather less likely than other schemes to report arrangements for care packaging by client subgroup, although the difference was not significant (Table 4.1). However, no case management schemes reported explicit targeting on elderly mentally infirm people.

This represents a serious failure to develop social work with demented elderly people. Bergmann, Foster, Justice and Matthews (1978) attempted to predict the destination of demented elderly people in different forms of household structure. They found first of all that demented elderly people living alone were least likely to remain at home over a period of one year despite the fact that this group attracted a greater flow of resources. Those living with a spouse were more likely to remain in the community, and those living with younger relatives most likely to.

So domiciliary resources should be concentrated on families caring for demented elderly people, although institutional care would often be the appropriate resource for the demented elderly living alone. For those dementing elderly people living with a spouse, a physical breakdown by the informal carer often played a part in precipitating a demand for institutional care. The relief of such burden on informal carers required much better care packaging than was evident. Challis

Table 4.1
Signs of efficiency improvement:
case management sector compared with
other sectors

Sign		Chi square	Direction
1.	Targeting (eligibility criteria)	2.45	positive
2.	Targeting (client subgroups)	2.15	negative
3.	Uptake	0.66	negative
4.	Outreach	1.05	negative
5.	Assessment (enhanced type)	0.46	positive
6.	Assessment (multidisciplinary)	9.32***	positive
7.	Care packaging	18.24***	positive
8.	Service arranging	47.72***	positive
9.	Direct work	9.47***	positive
10.	Monitoring/follow-up	6.65**	positive
11.	Key worker	37.19***	positive
12.	Personal care	1.22	negative
13.	Night sitting	1.53	negative
14.	Out-of-hours working	0.94	positive
15.	Short-term working	8.52***	positive
16.	Rehabilitation	10.42***	positive
17.	Shift from institutional care	0.01	negative
18.	Support for informal carers	0.01	positive
19.	More efficient production process	5.90**	positive
20.	Joint finance	2.10	negative
21.	Replication	1.59	positive
22.	Joint working with NHS	6.65***	positive

Notes
*   p at .10
**   p at .05
***   p at .01
Source: Ferlie et al. (1984).

and Davies (1986) outline some of the social work activities which could be undertaken in this setting: liaison with general practitioners to manage nocturnal restlessness, organising practical services or relief care as well as direct work such as providing an opportunity for the ventilation of feelings of guilt and anger. Vickery (1981) argues that many social workers fail to see these possibilities in their social work with old people, perceiving need instead in terms of provision of practical services: 'They were not only refraining from canvassing their skills as counsellors, resource finders, advocates, they were actively discouraging referrals for which their concrete services did not seem relevant.'

Horizontal target efficiency

Attempts to secure adequate inputs early in order to prevent rapid deterioration might be expected to be a feature of social work with elderly people and depend on adequate arrangements for case finding. The advocates of patch-based working (Hadley, Dale and Sills, 1984) argue that such community-centred teams would be more able to support informal carers and hence reduce crisis referrals. However, only eight of the 26 case management schemes reported enhanced uptake arrangements and although this was not significantly less than the rest of the sample (Table 4.1) there was certainly less emphasis than in the home help sector, where a majority of schemes reported such signs. The case management sector also performed poorly on other measures of horizontal target efficiency: only four schemes reported outreach activity, three an enhanced referral policy and five screening components.

Case management

This group of schemes above all others should pay most attention to case management. For example, without detailed assessment based on the examination of a range of needs rather than eligibility for isolated services, it will be difficult to construct effective care packages. Additionally, elderly people are likely to express by themselves very low levels of demand. So social workers may have to uncover hidden needs and perform a highly skilled diagnosis. Goldberg, Mortimer and Williams (1970) showed that unqualified social workers were less likely to report signs of depression in elderly clients than qualified social workers. Table 4.1, however, demonstrates that the case management sector was not significantly more likely than the rest of the sample to report enhancements in the type of assessment undertaken.

Only three schemes in the sector reported the use of new types of formal instrumentation in assessment procedures. For example, Essex's Alternatives to Residential Care Action Research Project provided an assessment document which specified the client's material or emotional problems and the caring tasks indicated. North Yorkshire's scale for assessing Part III residents covered physical disability, apathy, communication difficulty and disturbance. These projects were unusual in the sophistication of the assessment instrumentation employed.

The lack of depth and width in assessment means that requests for services are not examined fully nor alternatives considered nor explicit care plans capable of precise monitoring. Too often scarce resources silt up as a result of social workers taking out 'insurance policies' for their clients. Essex's Action Research Project on Part III Admissions (Ferlie, 1982) clearly shows the impact obtained from reviewing existing assessment procedures so as to force social workers to specify alternatives to residential care.

Assessment procedures may be improved in other ways. Awareness of the gap between staff, relatives' and clients' perceptions of the situation (Grad and Sainsbury, 1968) combined with the objective of supporting informal carers, has resulted in greater client or relative involvement in some assessment-based schemes. Carer perceptions must be taken seriously if management at home is to be considered as an option. For example, clients and relatives are involved in the initial case conference in Humberside's Rehabilitation Beds Scheme (Ferlie, 1982).

Table 4.1 shows that case management sector schemes are significantly more likely than other schemes to report multidisciplinary assessment procedures. Numerous studies have shown differences in assessments carried out on the same client by personnel with varying disciplinary backgrounds. Such differences are apparent between psychiatrists and social workers (Foster, Kay and Bergmann, 1976), between matrons of Part III homes and social workers (Plank, 1977) and between housing and social services department staff in allocating sheltered housing tenancies (Bytheway and James, 1978). In order to undertake broader assessment procedures, some innovators have developed multidisciplinary forms of assessment through joint visits, case conferences, or joint allocation panels.

A second question relates to the personnel involved in multidisciplinary assessment. Although schemes in the case management sector were significantly more likely to report multidisciplinary assessment than the rest of the sample, it was often multidisciplinary only in a rudimentary sense: home help organisers were much more likely to be reported to be making a joint assessment input alongside social workers (thirteen schemes) than health service professionals (only three reports were received of nursing input and two each of occupational therapist/physiotherapist input and consultant input). The crossing of agency boundaries is a major obstacle to the creation of effective case management procedures.

Attempts to establish care plans through negotiations with other agencies or sections on an *ad hoc* basis will often prove time-consuming and sometimes non-productive, especially if services operate with different models of care. A majority of schemes in the case management sector (fifteen) reported some care packaging functions, significantly more than in the rest of the sample (Table 4.1).

Some schemes specified in detail care packaging tasks undertaken. Three costed alternatives, the Kent Community Care Scheme using shadow prices which could 'cost' services bought in by social workers up to a global figure of two-thirds of the cost of a residential place. Five schemes reported tailoring packages of care to meet individual client needs, and seven reported interweaving with informal carers (out of the twelve in the whole sample reporting such tasks). The Oxford Community Care Project attempts to identify all existing formal and informal carers, establish their input and suggest modifications to their support if necessary. In Gateshead, strong family networks have meant that the Community Care Project there has put emphasis on working with families, to enable them to scale down their involvement to a manageable level.

These care plans involved a range of services: home help (twelve reports), Part III (eight reports), social work (six reports) and day care (five reports) were the services most often mentioned. Yet care packaging across conventional boundaries may face obstacles if decisions have to go up various line-management hierarchies. It is often difficult to introduce new forms of service arranging which broaden the roles of front-line workers and decentralise allocation decisions. Nevertheless, a majority of case management schemes reported moves towards improved service arranging (seventeen schemes), significantly more than the rest of the sample (Table 4.1). Often this was at the most basic level as more schemes reported enhanced negotiation procedures for services (seventeen) than a more radical change in prescriptive authority (five).

A number of techniques have been used in service arranging (Ferlie, 1982). The case conference system with key worker follow-up binds agencies *de facto* if not *de jure*. This may be SSD based (as in Cambridgeshire's Area Resource Panels) or joint (as in Bury's Beech Grove short-stay home). The 'core group' involved in this scheme consists of a range of SSD and NHS personnel, with a brief to make arrangements for post-discharge care as well as care within the home. A second option is to set up joint teams either within the boundaries of one agency or across agency boundaries. Brent has set up a specialist area team for the elderly, incorporating social work, domiciliary and other services. Some joint teams working across agency boundaries are able to prescribe a variety of services. The Oxfordshire Community Care Project, for example, consists of a senior social worker, a social worker, a district and a community psychiatric nurse and domiciliary care assistants. Such joint working can also proceed at a somewhat higher tier. The Isle of Wight Joint Care Planning Team (JCPT) set up an 'Elderly At Risk' group at nursing officer or team leader level able to prescribe a joint package of care. Officers are able to direct resources to meet needs within a yearly allocation not subject to fixed heads or *virement* procedures.

A distinction is conventionally drawn between the direct and case management roles of social workers, but innovations may advance along the two tracks simultaneously. Certainly the literature has criticised the frequent stereotyping of the problems of elderly people as simple (Parsloe and Stevenson, 1978) and points to family stress and feelings of bereavement, loss and isolation (Rowlings, 1981) which indicate a need for skilled social work involvement. Table 4.1 indicates that the schemes in the case management sector were significantly more likely to report direct work input: of the sixteen (out of 28) schemes that did so all reported direct work with elderly clients and six with relatives. A good example is the appointment of Durham's Senior Caseworker for the Elderly with a brief to develop intensive casework with families and individuals handling relationship work, bereavement and related emotional problems. However, few other schemes are as explicit in the development of direct work tasks.

The third stage of case management relates to monitoring, which enables workers not only to pick up changes in client need but also provides an instrument to combat social work 'drift'. Goldberg and Warburton's (1979) case review system embodied the specification of objectives and action plans as well as recording services and needs, reflecting a task-centred view of casework. However, only eight schemes in the case management sector reported the adoption of a monitoring system, although this was a significantly higher proportion than in the rest of the sample (Table 4.1). These monitoring systems were often in a rudimentary condition: only two specified set time intervals between reviews. So monitoring tasks represent a major area in which future development is required. Only six case management sector schemes reported arrangements for audit or review of performance and in all of these schemes internal rather than external scrutineers were involved. Only four schemes in the sector provided for an automatic case review on discharge from institutional care.

A further important 'sign' of case management is that of a key worker, defined by Goldberg and Connelly (1982) as incorporating case management and co-ordination functions as well as the monitoring role already outlined. Such brokerage and advocacy roles at front-line level take on great significance in a fragmented service system in which resource allocators higher up line management hierarchies may lack the information necessary to stitch together effective care packages. The Barclay Report (1982) also emphasised the indirect role that can be played by social workers in co-ordinating care services. Half the schemes in the case management sector reported a key worker system in operation, significantly more than the rest of the sample (Table 4.1).

However, the key worker functions reported centred more on the weaker term of 'co-ordination' (nine schemes) than the more precisely defined concepts of preparing papers for case conferences (three schemes), securing other services (five schemes) and monitoring (three schemes). Effective key workers may threaten other professionals' turf but the further development of a key worker system accords with the organisational imperatives of a fragmented, front-line-based service system. These key workers are overwhelmingly social workers (eleven of the twelve on which details were available in this sector) yet Goldberg and Warburton (1979) suggest that the social work culture has traditionally downgraded care packaging roles in favour of direct work, implying that the professional motivation for the effective development of key worker roles may not yet be present.

Service content

The sector performed well on indicators of case management. It is instructive to see whether this has been bought at the expense of enhancement of service content. Table 4.1 demonstrates that the sector was about as likely as the rest of the sample to report the achievement of three key signs of enhanced service content: personal care, night sitting and out-of-hours working. Although there is obviously less interest in these tasks, there does not appear to have been severe neglect.

Cost-related criteria

A major theme in social work with elderly people has been the development of short-term and task-centred casework. Reid and Shyne (1969) found that explicit short-term social work appeared to be more effective than long-term help among families with relationship difficulties. Goldberg and Connelly (1982, p.88) indicate how discrete task-centred casework could be applied to elderly people through enabling work, working through a period of mourning, easing relocation trauma or scaling down a excessive burden on carers through the construction of a care package of support.

Schemes in the case management sector were significantly more likely to provide for short-term working than the rest of the sample (Table 4.1). The short-term service offered was split evenly between post-hospital discharge work (four schemes), relief care (five schemes) and crisis work (four schemes) indicating that the move to a time-limited service does not just reflect domination by narrow bed-blocking criteria but more general preferences for a style of practice based on task-centred work and crisis intervention, often involving family support.

The sector also fared well in rehabilitative work. A number of institutional residents (Booth et al., 1982 suggest about 40 per cent of Part III residents are of low dependency) might have the potential for discharge given a transitional period of rehabilitation. The task of rehabilitation might be expected to be central to many care plans and indeed a clear majority of schemes in the sector reported rehabilitative work (twenty schemes), a significantly larger percentage than the rest of the the sample (Table 4.1). More reported an emphasis on physical rehabilitation (seven schemes) than other tasks: only one scheme reported the development of coping strategies or rehabilitation for elderly mentally infirm people as part of its brief. Even physical rehabilitative work, which may involve changes in an elderly person's home environment or routine, may be complex in terms of social work input. Such needs may not be readily perceived by elderly people, and Goldberg, Mortimer and Williams (1970, p.197) noted the importance of enabling work with elderly people, making needs explicit and helping clients to accept services to which they are entitled. Davies and Challis (1986, Chapter 6) point out that many elderly people may display anxiety about receiving help, fearing loss of autonomy. In such cases, social workers will have to work towards the provision of rehabilitative support at a pace which elderly people can accept.

The failure to develop social work with elderly mentally infirm people is particularly disturbing. Intervention with both the functionally mentally ill elderly and the demented would seem to warrant much greater priority. As far as the functionally ill are concerned, Kay, Beamish and Roth (1964) estimate the prevalence of depression and anxiety in the elderly population at about 28 per cent. Physical ill health and affective disorder are frequently associated (Roth and Kay, 1965). Post (1962) found that in only about 20 per cent of cases did depression in elderly people fail to respond to treatment. Yet existing services may fail to detect this morbidity: Bergmann's (1978) re-analysis of the Edinburgh study (Williamson et al., 1964) found that 61 per cent of neurotic and 71 per cent of depressive disorders were unknown to general practitioners.

Although a clear majority of case management schemes (twenty) reported a shift in the boundary from institutional to community care, this was almost exactly the same proportion as the sample as a whole. Nevertheless it is of interest that schemes emphasised the support of informal carers (ten schemes) suggesting a response to a perception of neglect in this field. Wenger (1982) has highlighted the inadequacy of social work support for informal carers, whereas Bayley and Parker's account (1980) of the Dinnington Project emphasises the poor links that exist between social workers and informal carers. However, the proportion of case management-based schemes offering support for informal carers was almost exactly the same as the sample as a whole (Table 4.1). Support offered included practical services such as domiciliary care (five schemes), day care (four schemes) and relief residential care (five schemes) as well as direct work with families, which was reported in six schemes. The rapid expansion of short-term residential care in recent years (Allen, 1982) has led to criticisms of the extra demands that higher resident throughput can place on care staff, but it should also be remembered that this service may be highly valued by relatives under stress.

Twelve case management schemes reported signs indicating a more efficient production process, a significantly higher proportion than the rest of the sample (Table 4.1). There was little concern with questions of economies or diseconomies of scale, rather emphasis was placed on improving the quality of work or management through training (four schemes) or enhanced management support (nine schemes). Bolton SSD has for example appointed a number of senior practitioners in the care of elderly people as consultants with a responsibility to develop services and train other team members. Note the reliance on developmental rather than line management-based attempts to alter patterns of front-line staff behaviour. The danger is that such consultancy roles, isolated from any power base within the organisation, remain marginal, with poor lines of communication down to practitioner level (Parsloe and Stevenson, 1978).

Finance

Table 4.1 demonstrates that case management-based schemes were somewhat less likely to receive joint finance than the rest of the sample, although the difference was not significant. However, whereas half the home help schemes received joint finance support, only a quarter of the case management-based schemes did so.

Continuing service differentiation raises a second question of service integration. The use of joint finance to fund case management systems which span agencies rather than service content-based innovations has not been a prominent theme. Only two reported schemes tackled cross-agency case management using joint finance. The Oxfordshire Community Care Project, led by a senior social worker, contains not only a social worker and domiciliary care assistants but also a district nurse and a community psychiatric nurse within a multidisciplinary team, although the team does not have direct access to hospital or

81

Part III facilities. The second example is Bolton's appointment of a senior social worker in a Multidisciplinary Assessment Team for the Elderly responsible for team co-ordination. The team includes a senior residential social worker, a nursing officer, a district nurse, a medical practitioner, a psychiatric nurse, an occupational therapist and physiotherapist. The team has control over six short-stay Part III assessment beds and access to four beds in the local hospital. Although these isolated developments are encouraging, it seems that the case management sector has made insufficiently creative use of joint finance.

Organisational process

Social work innovations could be thought to be more likely than innovations in basic services to result from a developmental model and less from environmental and budgetary shifts. The evidence on reported problem context offers some clues. Whereas in the home help sector about 60 per cent of schemes reported pressure on Part III beds as a reason for launching the innovation, in the case management sector this percentage fell to 40 per cent. Over half the schemes in the case management sector reported a developmental motive (the failure of existing services to meet needs as a reason for innovating), but 40 per cent of home help schemes also reported this. Hospital bed pressure was reported as a reason by about a quarter of schemes in both sectors. So there is no firm evidence to suggest that a developmental model of innovation fits case management innovation better than home help innovation.

A good example of a how a developmental model of innovation can also be linked to fears about misuse of scarce Part III resources is Essex's Action Research Project on Alternatives to Residential Care. This innovation attempted to develop social work skills with elderly people as a result of concerns that Part III waiting lists were being used by social workers as an insurance policy and did not reflect a true measure of need. Social workers were asked to undertake for those clients who would normally have been recommended Part III a more comprehensive assessment which specified the client's problems in terms of particular caring tasks and material or emotional problems. The project was, however, backed by management and the HQ-based research section and did not result from a 'bottom up' professionally-based process of innovation. Only rarely does it seem that front-line social workers (or indeed junior social work management) control the process of innovation within social work. Thus only one scheme in the case management sector was reported to have been initiated by social workers, as opposed to three by SSD senior management and four by a joint care planning team. This picture is in stark contrast to the process of innovation emerging in the NHS sector in which consultants were the group most often reported to be innovators. Other signs point to the marginality of many innovations in the sector: only four schemes reported a duration of more than five years, while only seven had extended their coverage to the whole of the local authority. The degree of replication, however, was not significantly different from that reported by the rest of the sample (Table 4.1). The picture appears to be one of centrally sponsored activity combining developmental and other reasons in which the localities have little say.

There are clearly boundaries to the pattern of lateral and inter-professional communication typical of case management schemes. Links with the NHS were reported in a majority of schemes (sixteen), a significantly higher proportion than the rest of the sample (Table 4.1). Poor formal interagency mechanisms of collaboration may be partially offset by good informal mechanisms and links with general practitioners were better developed than in the home help sector. However, only a small minority of schemes reported links with housing departments, voluntary organisations or indeed individual volunteers. Clearly the level of lateral communication undertaken by social workers has still to be developed fully in many innovations.

Discussion

The innovations reported in this sector were significantly more likely than the rest of the sample to display a number of key signs of case management. However, many were at a rudimentary stage of development with the result that when tight definitions of case management concepts were applied the number of schemes reporting such features fell sharply. But the sector was also significantly more likely to display some other efficiency signs such as short-term working.

It was disappointing to find the lack of SSD/NHS integrated case management, and especially the poor use of joint finance. Links with housing departments and the voluntary sector also seemed weak. Advances in service content did not go with advances in case management: the sector performed neither well nor badly on service content indicators. An important yet neglected model for development would be a joint NHS/SSD scheme which combined personal care support with a cross-agency case management system. Case management innovations have only begun to tackle some of these major issues.

The evidence also identified client subgroups where social work could be developed. Work with elderly mentally infirm people (both demented and depressed) was poorly articulated. There was little evidence of a substantial degree of direct work with informal carers through carer support groups. Social work with elderly people is but slowly developing the levels of skill which would enable it to shed its secondary status.

Case Studies

Gateshead Social Services Department Community Care Project

This scheme chose to expand the role of social work with elderly people through facilitating the extent of public sector entrepreneurial activity. Social workers were to co-ordinate and indeed create resources to be care packaged as well as undertaking counselling tasks. In addition care was made available to a wide variety of subgroups with special needs.

As Table 4.2 indicates, the scheme was aimed at those frail elderly at risk of admission to residential or hospital care but also included a concern for supporting families, by making their involvement manageable. Uptake was improved by the creation of new resources in care helpers (see Table 4.2), but otherwise stress was not laid on new case-finding devices.

Table 4.2
Gateshead SSD Community Care Project: case finding

Dimension	Response
Targeting (eligibility criteria)	On margin of need for residential care/frail
Targeting (client subgroups)	Elderly mentally infirm
	Stroke patients
	Incontinent
	Socially isolated
	Support for relatives
	Falls
	Elderly/physically handicapped
	Bereaved
Uptake	Intention to raise uptake by creation of more accessible resources
Outreach	No/no mention
Mandatory assessment	General commitment
Preventive surveillance	Good neighbours
	SSD staff

As Table 4.3 makes clear, improved case management is one of the main aspects of the scheme. Each client is fully assessed to ascertain problems, including an appraisal of help received from informal carers. Thorough care planning functions are promoted: there is a decentralised budget, tailoring and emphasis on supporting informal carers. Although social workers are not able to allocate other resources (except for voluntary care helpers) directly, they can influence the allocation of home help hours as part of establishing a care plan. They also undertake direct work with carers as well as counselling and groupwork sessions as a form of localised day care. All of the work done by the team is monitored both in terms of effects on clients and costs. The level and nature of care provided can be modified in line with any changes in the client's circumstances.

Clients receive both domestic and personal care, with flexible hours. The scheme has been able to cater for the special needs of elderly mentally infirm people, the socially isolated and physically frail as well as the initial target group (see Table 4.4).

Table 4.5 outlines various ways in which service efficiency can be measured. The scheme was designed to provide a crisis intervention service in which intensive services could be provided for a short period and then withdrawn. The scheme offered rehabilitative support for the physically frail and the depressed, together with the provision of management for the demented. Much of this work was undertaken by volunteers, working at a high level of skill, which together with other scheme resources was aimed at reducing the burden on informal carers. The provision of small local day centres represented a new low-cost resource. The project was funded by Inner Areas Project (IAP) money for an initial period of three years.

As Table 4.6 indicates, the scheme sprang out of a concern about inflexible responses to growing pressures on Part III beds. External finance was required and the project was launched through top management IAP bids for a pilot scheme to run in half the borough, with the eastern area forming a control area. It was essentially an internal SSD initiative. It is therefore perhaps not surprising that enhanced liaison with other agencies was not reported (see Table 4.7). Indeed the care helpers were the resource with which the most substantial joint working was undertaken.

The scheme was evaluated by a research officer linked to the University of Kent.

Conclusion The scheme produced advances in both counselling and care packaging functions. The development of relationship work with a traditionally neglected client group went hand in hand with the co-ordination and development of resources.

Table 4.3
Gateshead SSD Community Care Project:
case management

Dimension	Response
Assessment (type)	Focus on problems/strengths rather than eligibility for service
	Formal instrumentation used: schedules for physical capacity, mental state and social support
Assessment (inputs)	Social workers
	Nursing staff
	OTs/physiotherapists
	GPs
	Clients' significant others/informal carers
Care packaging (type)	Account taken of varying costs of alternatives
	Prescribed budgetary limits
	Tailoring
	Emphasis on supporting/increasing inputs from informal carers
Care packaging (scope)	SSD domiciliary care
	SSD day care
	SSD residential care
	SSD fieldwork services
	NHS community services
	Voluntary inputs
Arranging for additional services	Negotiating procedure for arranging other services by the SSD
	Power to purchase private/voluntary services
	Contractual arrangements, e.g. for informal helpers
Direct work	With client
	With other informal carers
Monitoring (type)	Set time intervals
Monitoring (scope)	SSD domiciliary care
	SSD day care
	SSD fieldwork services
	NHS community services
	NHS day hospitals
	Informal inputs
Monitoring (by whom?)	Social workers
	Community nurses
Audit/review?	Set time period: six months or less
Key worker (role)	Co-ordination
	Implementing care plan
Key worker (who?)	Social workers
	Community nurses
Post-institutional care review	No/no mention

Table 4.4
Gateshead SSD Community Care Project:
care provision

Dimension	Response
Personal care	General commitment
Domestic care	General commitment
Night sitting	Yes
Out-of-hours working	Yes
Specialist care (eligibility criteria)	On margin of need for institutional care
Specialist care (client subgroups)	Elderly mentally infirm
	Socially isolated
	Support for relatives
	Elderly/physically handicapped

Table 4.5
Gateshead SSD Community Care Project:
efficiency

Dimension	Response
Short-term commitment	Relief care
Rehabilitation	Physical rehabilitation
	EMI coping strategies
	Incontinence
	Emotional support for anxiety/depression
Lower-cost mode	Shift from institutional care
	Support for informal carers
	Use of volunteers
Support for informal carers	Domiciliary care
	Day care
	Volunteers
More efficient production process	Removal of diseconomies of scale
Source of finance	SSD base budget
	Inner Areas Project

Table 4.6
Gateshead SSD Community Care Project:
organisational process

Dimension	Response
Problem context	Observed failure of present service. disregard of client preferences and excessive rigidity Pressure on OPH beds Demographic trends
Initiating personnel	SSD individual senior managers
Pilot?	Yes
Duration	Less than 5 years
Coverage	Several districts

Table 4.7
Gateshead SSD Community Care Project:
joint working

Dimension	Response
Joint working (NHS staff)	Nurses GPs Physiotherapists
Joint working (housing department staff)	No/no details
Individual volunteers	General commitment
Voluntary organisations	No/no details
New forms of internal cross working	No/no details
Evaluation (by implementors)	No/no details
Evaluation (by other internal officers)	No/no details
Evaluation (by external evaluators)	University departments/units

Isle of Wight Social Services Department Joint Care of the Elderly 'At Risk'

This scheme was set up to promote joint working between all agencies concerned with elderly people 'at risk', based mainly at team leader/

nursing officer level. It included representatives of the voluntary sector. Because it included health inputs a slightly expanded coding frame was devised covering health care.

The group was aimed at ensuring that elderly persons in the community at risk of gradual or imminent collapse receive the fullest help possible (see Table 4.8). One of the main tasks was to identify frail or isolated elderly people unknown to agencies and then to persuade such elderly people that help could prolong their life at home. The joint nature of the group simplified the referral process. One of the voluntary groups represented ran a street link scheme for monitoring elderly people so that preventive surveillance could be undertaken.

Care planning functions were prominent. The budget was flexible so that others could direct resources to meet individual needs within a yearly allocation not subject to fixed headings and normal *virement* procedures. The group, comprising social work team leaders, community nursing officers, domiciliary services officers, voluntary organisations and specialist consultants, were called upon as appropriate. In addition to these arrangements, short-term admissions to private and voluntary homes were (unusually) available. As Table 4.9 indicates, each elderly person was monitored until the presenting need no longer arose, or a long-term review process was instituted. The group could also decide to withdraw services if this was unwarranted. Each client was allocated a key worker with responsibility for implementing the care plan and providing feedback.

A variety of inputs could be deployed: domiciliary physiotherapy

Table 4.8
Isle of Wight SSD Joint Care
of the Elderly At Risk:
case finding

Dimension	Response
Targeting (eligibility criteria)	On margin of need for residential care
Targeting (client subgroups)	No/no mention
Uptake	No such intention/mention
Outreach	Elderly/physically handicapped Socially isolated
Referral process	More direct access to services
Preventive surveillance	Good neighbours

Table 4.9
Isle of Wight SSD Joint Care
of the Elderly At Risk:
case management

Dimension	Response
Assessment (type)	No/no mention
Assessment (inputs)	No/no mention
Care packaging (type)	Account taken of varying costs of alternatives
	Prescribed budgetary limits
Care packaging (scope)	SSD domiciliary care
	SSD day care
	SSD residential care
	SSD fieldwork services
	NHS community services
	NHS hospitals
	Other housing services (not sheltered housing)
	Voluntary inputs
Arranging for additional services	Innovation in formal procedure by the SSD and by other agencies for arranging other services
	Power to purchase private/voluntary services
Direct work	No/no mention
Monitoring (type)	General commitment
Monitoring (scope)	General commitment
Monitoring (by whom?)	General commitment
Audit/review?	General commitment
Key worker (role)	Implementing care plan
	Monitoring
Key worker (who?)	General commitment

(to aid mobility), home help and community nursing. Some of the volunteers (Red Cross, Cancer Relief) offered skills in dealing with medical conditions. Many of the elderly people helped were either isolated or physically handicapped, posing extra demands on the scheme (see Table 4.10).

The scheme was able to offer various kinds of short-term support (see Table 4.11). As well as boarding out and short-term admissions to residential care, the group was able to co-ordinate resources to provide 24-hour care at home for a limited period in emergencies. Although many elderly people require help so that they can remain

Table 4.10
Isle of Wight SSD Joint Care
of the Elderly At Risk:
care provision

Dimension	Response
Enhanced physical facilities	General commitment
Domestic care	General commitment
Personal care	General commitment
Nursing care	General commitment
Specialist care (eligibility criteria)	On margin of need for institutional care Insufficient informal carers
Specialist care (client subgroups)	Socially isolated Elderly/physically handicapped

Table 4.11
Isle of Wight SSD Joint Care
of the Elderly At Risk:
efficiency

Dimension	Response
Short-term commitment	Relief care Crisis work
Rehabilitation	Social skills/independence Physical rehabilitation
Lower-cost mode	Shift from institutional care Support for informal carers Use of volunteers
Support for informal carers	Relief residential care
More efficient production process	No/no mention
Source of finance	Joint finance

at home until they die, a domiciliary physiotherapy service is available to promote physical rehabilitation. In other cases, social integration has been stressed so as to improve conditions at home. A move away from unnecessary residential care has thus been promoted by the introduction of a more co-ordinated and systematic approach to community care, by support for informal carers and by the use of volunteers. The initial joint funding budget of £123,000 was later increased to £155,000.

As Table 4.12 makes clear, the mechanism behind the scheme lay in the decision in 1979 of the Joint Care Planning Team, in view of the needs of the Isle of Wight's increasing elderly population (proportionally one of the highest in the country) and to reduce pressure on overloaded residential facilities. The joint group was co-chaired by a specialist in community medicine and a SSD assistant director operating across the whole of the Island. The former also acted as the link with the housing department.

As well as a well developed pattern of liaison with other agencies, community development (see Table 4.13) was promoted in the sense that a new voluntary fund was set up as a financial supplement. As far as evaluation was concerned, it was hoped to involve researchers from Southampton University.

Conclusion This scheme represents a well-developed attempt to improve liaison between agencies at decision-making level. The group was given executive responsibility to arrange a wide variety of resources.

Table 4.12
Isle of Wight SSD Joint Care
of the Elderly At Risk:
organisational process

Dimension	Response
Problem context	Pressure on OPH beds
	Demographic trends
Initiating personnel	Joint working: JCPT/top tier initiative
Pilot?	No/no mention
Duration	Less than 5 years
Coverage	Authority-wide

Table 4.13
Isle of Wight SSD Joint Care
of the Elderly At Risk:
joint working

Dimension	Response
Joint working (SSD staff)	General commitment
Joint working (NHS staff)	General commitment
Joint working (volunteers/ voluntary organisations)	Local charities Red Cross
Joint working (housing department staff)	General commitment
Community development	Creation of new voluntary resources
Evaluation (by implementors)	No/no details
Evaluation (by other internal officers)	No/no details
Evaluation (by external evaluators)	Yes

5 Innovation in Other SSD Support Services

Commentary

This chapter analyses 47 innovations reported in Ferlie, Challis and Davies (1983) comprising all those schemes launched by SSDs not already discussed in Chapters 3 and 4. These services consist of assisted lodging schemes (fifteen reports), day care (thirteen reports), short-term care (six reports), community care groups (six reports), new forms of residential support (three schemes), street wardens (three schemes) and relative support schemes (two reports). Due to the very disparate nature of the sector, the three main groups of schemes reported will be examined separately. This cuts down the numbers in each category and therefore no statistical tests of significance were employed in this chapter. Detailed examples are again taken from Ferlie (1982).

Assisted lodgings

In assisted lodgings schemes accommodation is arranged by a voluntary or statutory agency with a host who is usually expected to provide more care and support than is usual in a landlady/tenant relationship. The extent of care, the length of stay and the degree of dependency catered for will of course vary. Some schemes cater for elderly clients solely but others serve a mixture of client groups. The function of these schemes also varies considerably: some lodgings represent a form of holiday relief care for relatives more acceptable to old people than short stay in Part III, others offer a base for convalescence or a permanent home for elderly people who have spent many years in hospital but could be discharged to a supportive environment.

Assisted lodgings schemes expanded rapidly in the 1970s. Thornton and Moore (1980) could identify only 23 current schemes which placed elderly people in private households. They estimated that only about 50 elderly people were in long-term placements at the end of April 1980 and that about 285 clients had short stays in 1979. Thornton and Moore concluded that there was scope for service extension and for securing a greater degree of service variety in meeting needs. Considerable further growth is evident since 1980.

Voluntary organisation-based assisted lodgings schemes for elderly people first emerged in the 1950s and by the 1960s were well established in some areas. The National Old People's Welfare Council found in 1965 that 50 respondent committees had some sort of boarding-out scheme. They were often run by Old People's Welfare Committees or Councils of Voluntary Service and the larger schemes could place on average 30–40 people a year. The new schemes which emerged in the 1970s differed in a number of key respects from the earlier model (Thornton and Moore, 1980, p.22): they were smaller-scale, they were more likely to be run by the SSD, they faced an issue of increased client dependency, they used private households in a greater variety of ways, they provided more social work support and they paid 'fees' to carers. The pressure to develop such resources further sprang most often from pressure on conventional Part III and hospital provision and the desire to provide relief care for relatives.

Vertical target efficiency A number of vertical targeting difficulties were reported in Thornton and Moore's review of assisted lodgings schemes. As far as short-term schemes were concerned, some agencies had not found it easy to state explicit objectives and define specific client groups. In some cases, a short-term service developed as an unplanned consequence of carers offering such support in response to publicity aimed at recruiting carers for longer-term support. In long-term schemes the scarcity of carers may mean that their preferences are accorded priority over client needs. Schemes will also often place restrictions on the degree of dependency that may be handled. There is general agreement that a client should not require 'nursing care', although care that 'a relative might be expected to give' (presumably personal care) is included as a requirement in some projects. Other conditions not tolerated by schemes frequently include dementia and incontinence.

On the other hand, Ferlie, Challis and Davies (1983) indicate tight targeting around administratively defined eligibility criteria: eleven of the fifteen assisted lodgings schemes reported targeting by eligibity criteria. These schemes all employed concepts of frail/Part III marginal (six reports) or post-hospital discharge (five reports) as means of targeting. There were fewer reports of targeting by client subgroup criteria. Of the six such reports, five related to relative support.

Horizontal target efficiency Thornton and Moore (1980) report that in some schemes it had proved difficult to 'find' enough clients. Whereas it proved relatively easy to identify mentally ill elderly people living in hospital, it proved much more problematic to identify elderly people in Part III or the community who could benefit from the assisted lodgings programme. Indeed some of those who could benefit from the service are socially isolated, with poor social networks which could not be tapped for referral. There are also difficulties in some schemes in persuading social workers (who will not usually be specialists in the care of elderly people) of the value of the scheme, a difficulty encountered in many specialist services dependent on referral from generic workers. In part also there was a conflict between the immediate demands of front-line social workers for action in a crisis and the aim of many adult fostering schemes for careful preparatory work and matching.

Ferlie, Challis and Davies (1983) confirm the argument that assisted lodgings schemes often exhibit little concern for horizontal target efficiency. No scheme reported the use of mandatory assessment or preventive surveillance activities or the performing of measures designed to increase uptake. Only two schemes undertook outreach activity. The impression is of a cluster of schemes reluctant to excite demand if only because of tight constraints on 'supply', that is the number of families willing to offer care. Outreach activity might rather be concentrated among carers than clients. Thornton and Moore (1980) argue that although some schemes have remained small-scale resources, the reason for this reflects inadequate recruitment campaigns rather than structural obstacles. Carers were able to cope with quite high degrees of client dependency: in their analysis of short-term provision, they found that two-thirds of carers had helped with bathing. There may well be scope for more effective outreach activity designed to recruit additional carers.

Case management At least some of the recent assisted lodgings schemes operate with a fostering and adoption model in which great stress is placed on social work assessment, matching and support (Thornton and Moore, 1980). Nearly half the schemes (seven)

96

reported an emphasis on assessment, although in only one case was this undertaken on a multidisciplinary basis. In the majority of cases a social worker undertook the assessment task. However, other essential tasks of case management were less well represented. The impression that many assisted lodgings schemes act as a discrete alternative to other forms of provision was reinforced by the lack of reports of arrangements for care planning (one scheme) or service arranging (one scheme). Thornton and Moore (1980, p.143) comment that some schemes made provision in their original designs for carers to receive domiciliary or day care relief as appropriate, but in practice provision is rarely made.

It was, however, noteworthy that eight schemes provided for a direct work service, which could be undertaken either with elderly clients or the caring family. In particular matching activity emerged as an important social work task in fostering-oriented schemes, although in more traditional boarding-out schemes carers were found to be more intolerant of delays possibly for financial reasons. Such mechanisms as introductory visits and trial weekends were found to reassure many clients. In some schemes (such as Camden's Adult Care Scheme) the introduction to assisted lodgings can spread over a period of months.

Only one scheme reported monitoring activity. None reported provision for an audit of resources or the appointment of a key worker. However, eight schemes reported the provision of personal care tasks (such as bathing and dressing) confirming the view that carers were able to cope with clients of high as well as slight physical dependency.

Cost-related criteria Assisted lodgings schemes performed well on many of the technical efficiency signs employed. However, the more fostering-oriented schemes will also involve a considerable amount of skilled social work time in assessment and support. The initial costs of vetting carers and setting up placements are high but diminish if a stable body of carers can be found and bonding established between carers and clients who require intermittent care.

Eleven schemes reported provision for a short-term service, concentrated in relief care work (seven reports) rather than post-hospital discharge care, post-Part III discharge care or crisis intervention (one report each). Thornton and Moore's discussion (1980, p.67) of the wide range of potential objectives of short-term assisted lodgings schemes reflects initial hopes rather than operational details. In practice short-term care schemes have been heavily targeted on the relief of relatives, and other functions have not been so well developed.

A majority of schemes also reported rehabilitative working (nine reports), especially the provision of emotional support for anxiety or depression, neglected in other sectors. In some cases clients are likely to have been socially isolated, although others will be moving from institutional care. For example, Barnet's Adult Boarding Out Scheme (Ferlie, 1982) makes provision for several types of service, including family care, which offers not only accommodation but also the provision of reassurance and encouragement for adults (not just elderly people) who are trying to regain independence. The historic link in boarding-out schemes between provision for the mentally ill and rehabilitative activity was evident in this scheme.

In view of the weak links with ex-Part III clients, it was surprising that all fifteen schemes claimed to be pursuing a lower cost mode through providing alternatives to institutional care. Schemes seemed to act more as preventive rather than post-discharge resources. In order to qualify for the Salop Boarding Out Scheme (Ferlie, 1982) an elderly person must be in need of care and attention that would not otherwise be available and be on the waiting list for Part III accommodation. Eight schemes reported support for relatives as a means of reducing pressure on Part III, through the provision of a relief service. Thornton and Moore (1980, pp.96-7) comment that relatives approached in the course of their study appeared to have confidence in the efficiency of the scheme and the capabilities of the carers. However, there was often little evaluation of whether such relief care improved the quality of the relationship between the relative and the elderly person. In some cases, the relationship appeared to become more strained after the return home when the elderly person unfavourably compared the care and attention offered with that received during the placement.

Only two schemes reported training for carers. The Leeds scheme provides for three or four half-day meetings for carers each year together with an annual three-day training session. However, if schemes are expected to cater for clients of at least moderate dependency, increased training may become necessary. Thornton and Moore (1980, p.141) argue that it may be a mixed blessing that many carers tend to have nursing backgrounds: engrained knowledge may sometimes have to be unlearnt if it is dependency-inducing.

The possibility of utilising joint finance for assisted lodgings schemes has been mentioned (Thornton and Moore, 1980, p.161). However, the schemes were mainly SSD base budget based (eleven reports) with joint finance (three reports) playing a minor role. This pattern of funding could well be associated with the weak links with post-institutional care.

Organisational process Assisted lodgings schemes are undertaken in response to a variety of problems: failures in existing services (four reports), awareness of demographic pressure (two reports) but most importantly pressure on institutional facilities (nine reports). Although in other contexts stress on the relief of pressure on institutional care is associated with a 'top down approach', in this sector a 'bottom up' approach is more favoured, with social work practitioners taking on initiating roles. In the case of fostering-oriented schemes, social work skills represent the crucial technology transfer from the child care field to work with elderly people. In other cases schemes have expanded incrementally, often from a mental health base, as social workers have sought to extend the range of facilities available. Bottom-up innovation displays acute problems of marginality: eleven schemes had been in operation for less than five years and although coverage was often authority-wide the volume of work undertaken was small. There were poor lines of communication with other agencies: liaison with housing departments or the NHS was rarely mentioned (one report each), although links with voluntary organisations were almost as poor (two reports).

Thornton and Moore (1980, p.173) acknowledge that the emergence of fostering with elderly people can justly be described as an innovative development but go on to criticise an unimaginative approach to implementation. Certainly more schemes should develop a greater variety of approaches, as some (for example Camden's Adult Care Programme) have already done. This section has drawn attention to other fundamental problems such as lack of integration both at client and organisational levels. The negative consequences of this have included poor care planning at client level and poor relationships between specialist and front-line teams which have led to difficulties in securing referrals. The brief of assisted lodgings schemes has also often been narrowly interpreted to mean relief for relatives. Above all there is the problem of scale. Only a couple of schemes reported development from experimental resources to significant mainstream projects. Thornton and Moore (1980, p.164) speculate that the worsened financial climate has made life more difficult for such projects. This argument could be developed further: a colder financial climate will hit especially hard bottom-up innovations without powerful central sponsors or access to external sources of funding.

Day care

The National Assistance Act of 1948 empowered local authorities to provide social activities for the handicapped where care and social activities might take place, this discretionary power becoming mandatory in 1960. This power was widened by the 1962 National Assistance

Amendment Act which empowered local authorities to provide meals and recreation for elderly people and to make use of voluntary bodies as their agents. Carter (1981, p.28) estimates that the voluntary sector provides 57 per cent of the day care provision for elderly people in England and Wales. In this section public sector provision only is considered, as voluntary sector day care provision will be analysed in Chapter 8.

Despite rapid expansion, a number of key problems have been identified with the service. One is poor targeting: what is day care meant to achieve for whom? A second concern is fear of poor service content in that day care has often been seen as dull and as taking place in inadequate premises. Carter (1981, p.37) found that only 5 per cent of day care units for elderly people offered an educational programme and only one in seven organised meetings and discussion groups. A third problem is the availability and cost of transport. Two-thirds of day hospitals in Carter's study (1981, p.43) complained of problems in timing the service to meet transport timetables and the patients' convenience. As far as cost is concerned, Fennell, Emerson, Sidell and Hague (1981) estimate that transport constitutes about a quarter of the total costs of the service. A final area of concern is that very few members of staff in day care settings possess professional qualifications as it is essentially a lay service. Goldberg and Connelly (1982, p.131) comment on the basis of previous day care studies that staff who have had training expressed interest in further training, whereas those with no training experience did not. It seemed that organisers were often left to their own devices on appointment and appeared to be isolated from other service providers. It was perhaps because of these difficulties that Carter (1981, p.40) found only a 70 per cent occupancy in the units for elderly people studied, despite recurrent reports of pressure on day hospital places. Day care is a service which has enjoyed a period of quantitative expansion but which is now faced with important organisational and service content problems.

Vertical target efficiency Within the spectrum of day care there is a continuum ranging from unallocated places in 'pop in' day care, through allocated day care places to day hospital places. There is evidence to suggest that the allocation of this variety of day care places is often badly matched to needs. This may be because there is a deliberate policy to mix elderly people of different types, although Fennell et al. (1981) recommend an allocation policy based on client group homogeneity as helpful to new users.

Where targeting by dependency level is accepted as a policy, it is useful to recall Goldberg and Connelly's argument (1982, p.122) that appropriate users of day services fall into five categories: (i) the reasonably well and active who go to drop in centres or lunch clubs for social or preventive reasons; (ii) the isolated or depressed elderly in need of a social stimulus; (iii) those who would benefit medically from day hospital services; (iv) the physically disabled who need social support and where relatives might also require relief care; and (v) the confused or mentally ill, especially those living with stressed relatives.

Targeting arrangements are frequently less well defined in practice. Edwards, Sinclair and Gorbach (1980) suggest that the more dependent elderly who require transport receive less day care than the fitter elderly who do not. Day care by itself may be inadequate to meet care objectives. Fennell et al. (1981) suggest that day care alone will not achieve reduction of relative stress to manageable levels, although Arie (1975) questions the assumption that day care can manage the severely elderly mentally infirm. As far as day hospital places are concerned, Brocklehurst (1979) argues that the development of the service has been retarded because many patients come for maintenance or social support rather than active medical input. Hildick-Smith (1980) draws attention to the effects of a lack of day centre places on the way in which a day hospital can operate, making it difficult to discharge treated but isolated patients.

Precisely targeted allocation depends on well developed assessment procedures. Yet the assessment procedures in many day centres for elderly people described by Carter (1981, p.33) are rudimentary. Units often operated with an inverse 'eligibility criteria' model which ensured that the greater the need, the less likely an elderly person was to get a place. Examples of such inverse eligibility criteria include the presence of disruptive behaviour, incontinence or dementia. Of the thirteen public sector day care schemes in Ferlie, Challis and Davies (1983), only two reported targeting by administrative criteria, namely marginality to entry to or discharge from institutional care. Eight schemes reported targeting by subgroup characteristics, most usually confusion, relatives' stress or physical dependency. The Leicestershire day centre schemes represent good examples (Ferlie, 1982) of schemes catering for higher levels of physical dependency than is usual. Yet five schemes reported no targeting policy at all, illustrating the danger that day care is often provided without a clear idea of objectives or target clienteles.

Horizontal target efficiency Some of the aims often associated with day care intervention (such as relief of stressed relatives or the provision of company for the socially isolated) might be associated with an emphasis on horizontal target efficiency. Schemes designed to increase horizontal target efficiency also tackle the key problem of transport through a number of devices. Mobile day centres are a way of bringing day care to elderly people in rural communities: an example in Sunderland examined by Kaim-Caudle (1977) aimed at elderly people of moderate dependency proved itself to be an economic and acceptable service. Projects such as the Gateshead Community Care Scheme (Ferlie, 1982) have provided new forms of local day care in informal settings. Certainly a number of the day care schemes reported uptake (six reports) and outreach (five reports) activity. For example, the Southwark Day Centre for the Elderly Mentally Infirm places emphasis on drawing relatives into resource centre-based forms of support:

> In addition to activities for the users, the involvement of families will be encouraged. Lack of contact between families and staff can result in misunderstanding on both sides. The staff may see the family as having 'dumped' their elderly relative, whereas the families may see the staff as controlling and interfering. Contact with the family is therefore very important, and attendance at a regular relatives group will be encouraged (Ferlie, 1982, p.149).

Case management Goldberg and Connelly (1982, pp.133–4) argue that poor case management is likely to be a besetting sin of much day care work, reflecting organisational discontinuities both between the NHS and the SSD and within different sections of the SSD itself. There is likely to be poor liaison with external agencies, little emphasis on record keeping or monitoring, and little service co-ordination. Additional weaknesses include social workers withdrawing from cases once day care has been allocated, little interweaving with relatives and poor co-ordination with the domiciliary services. Although Fennell et al. (1981) report that 42 per cent of day centre attenders were also in receipt of home help, they were not able to present evidence about the extent of liaison between the two services.

The report on MIND's Sheffield scheme illustrates the difficulties day care centres face in interweaving with the relatives of elderly mentally infirm people and of involving voluntary sources of care:

> the initial idea was that relatives might well wish to help in a day centre, in exchange for time off from their own relatives. It was also felt that there would be enough voluntary help for it to be a community based scheme. Neither of these expectations was realised. The terrible pressure on relatives necessitated their being offered time off with no strings attached, while local volunteers have been difficult to recruit . . . Volunteers often felt despondent due to the lack of signs of visible success and were unable to provide a reliable service (Ferlie, 1982, p.474).

Of the thirteen entries in the day centre category (Ferlie, Challis and Davies, 1983), only four reported explicit assessment (usually in those schemes catering for higher need groups such as elderly mentally infirm people) and one care planning. This scheme was Haringey's Woodside Club Psychogeriatric Centre (Ferlie, 1982, p.145) where explicit decisions had been made to increase staffing levels and to introduce new proposals following the retirement of the previous officer-in-charge. The centre's new aims included initial assessment of client needs, in conjunction with other workers, and the development of a care plan and the introduction of regular reassessments to monitor changes in the state of clients' health. Such case management was exceptional, however: no schemes reported service arranging features. Three schemes reported direct work. The Highbury Day Centre for the Elderly Mentally Infirm (Ferlie, 1982, p.157) emphasised the stimulation of intellectual activity and help with maintaining or relearning daily living skills, but such work was uncommon. Further signs of case management were equally neglected. Only two schemes reported monitoring systems and none the appointment of a key worker. This lack of case management is a serious weakness of the day care sector and stems from the acceptance of modest custodial objectives. As Fennell et al. conclude:

> Organisers are generally left to their own devices on appointment and assistants are simply shown their duties on the job. While good results may be obtained in this way it is symptomatic of the modest goals held by policy makers for day centres and restricts the spread of imaginative ideas which individual organisers may have (Fennell et al., 1981, p.206).

There are a number of ways in which case management could be improved. For example, Fennell et al. (1981) found that domiciliary visits to assess the home situation were often not officially encouraged within day care settings, as being outside the range of day care organiser duties.

Cost-related criteria One of the effects of a poor assessment and monitoring procedure is a failure to develop means of controlling case flow on a systematic basis. Goldberg and Connelly (1982, p.134) argue that client reviews are especially important given a combination of low occupancy rates, waiting lists and lack of liaison between the day care and day hospital sectors over transfer. Assessment and allocation for a defined short-term service would in these circumstances seem a difficult task: it is not surprising that only two schemes report a short-term service.

There is, however, a substantial stress on rehabilitation reported of these innovations. This contrasts with Carter's (1981, p.205) finding that in the day care sector as a whole rehabilitation was not emphasised. In her sample, only one in seven of responding staff thought rehabilitation to be an aim of the unit, these units being more likely to be those serving the mentally ill. In day centres for elderly people, diversionary activity was emphasised at the expense of a rehabilitative function: a likely consequence of a lay service. However, eight of the thirteen schemes in Ferlie, Challis and Davies (1985) reported rehabilitative work ranging from stimulating elderly mentally infirm people, to ensuring the availability of medical services within day care settings catering for more physically handicapped elderly people.

This sharpening of purpose was also evident in reports concerning moves towards a lower cost mode for service. The model for day care based on providing companionship for the socially isolated was less common than that which stressed the role of day care in avoiding recourse to institutional care (eleven reports), support for informal carers (seven reports) and the use of volunteers (three reports). The extent to which these services succeed in relieving relatives is an important issue. Small-scale evaluation projects connected with the Buckinghamshire Park Club (Chisholm and Fletcher, 1979) and a Sheffield MIND Project (Mendel, 1979) have examined the impact of day care for elderly mentally infirm people on stressed relatives and concluded on the basis of carer interviews that a substantial degree of carer relief was achieved, even if the degree of client confusion could not be reduced. Both studies also concluded that there was a need for social work support, particularly in cases of continuing deterioration which could result in placement in residential care.

A further development is the increasing involvement of joint finance in day care innovations: eight of the thirteen schemes reported joint finance input, whereas six reported SSD base budget input. What are the likely repercussions of this shift in the method of financing? Jointly financed day care innovations were more likely to cater for the more dependent groups (such as the demented or physically dependent) where there was emphasis on preventing institutionalisation.

Organisational process Carter (1981, p.326) clearly sees day care units as a 'bottom-up' system, where developmental initiative is assumed to lie at front-line level. Thus Carter argues that heads of establishments should place greater emphasis on communicating 'upwards' about priorities and development. Additionally, the note of isolation she detected in some of the facilities was seen as due to over-long chains of managerial accountability. Reports on initiating personnel were available on only eight schemes, which is insufficient for firm conclusions. Of these eight, four reported the involvement solely of front-line workers in the innovatory process, although four reported the involvement of higher tier officers. Certainly the increasing involvement of joint finance and tightening of objectives could imply a shift from bottom-up to top-down innovation within the sector.

Day care innovations are also likely to exhibit signs of marginality. Only two had lasted for longer than five years, and only one had been replicated. The replication of innovations where both new staff attitudes and new sites are required may be considerably more difficult than replication of innovations in the domiciliary and social work sectors where only changes to service approach are required. Although schemes were likely to report relatively good links with voluntary resources (nine reports), links with other sections of the SSD or other public agencies were less well developed. Thus six schemes reported links with the NHS, two with housing departments and only one reported close working relationships with social workers. This was the Southwark Day Centre for the Elderly Mentally Infirm which, in a neat inversion of usual roles, was seen as a teaching centre for social workers and other professionals who could learn from the specialist expertise of the Centre staff.

In conclusion, many of the conventional criticisms of day care provision can equally be applied to day care innovations: there is moderate emphasis only on vertical target efficiency and poor case management. There is a continuing note of isolation about many of the facilities. Yet there are also countervailing pressures. The desire to use day care in a more focused way to prevent unnecessary institutional care and relieve stressed relatives is associated with the utilisation of joint finance and possibly increased 'top down' interest in sector development.

New forms of residential care

There are nine schemes in this subcategory (Ferlie, Challis and Davies, 1983), consisting of schemes based on relief, rotating or intermittent care (six schemes) and those which are based on a support unit concept (three schemes).

Allen (1982) points to the rapid growth in the use of short-term residential care for elderly people in recent years. Although only 2 per cent of beds in Part III were designated for short-stay purposes in 1980, they accounted for some 60 per cent of admissions, as opposed to only 30 per cent in 1967. Short-stay care is mainly provided in residential homes predominantly occupied by long-term residents, rather than specialist short-stay homes. The functions as well as the scale of the programme have undergone a process of expansion. Whereas short-stay care was initially designed to allow carers to go on holiday, it now covers a much broader spread of needs, including a holiday for elderly clients, convalescence, assessment, preparation for a permanent Part III admission, or short-term relief for stressed carers. In addition, whereas short-stay care was originally defined as two or three weeks once a year, it is sometimes now offered on a rotating or intermittent basis. Allen (1982) also discusses some of the disadvantages that the increase in the short-stay programme has had in terms of extra demands on home management. For some establishments extra confused or physically handicapped short-stay admissions could make the difference between coping and not coping. Heads running group unit homes found it particularly difficult to fit short-stay residents into groups, and long-term residents often had little to do with short-stay residents. Short-term residents themselves could find frequent moves disorientating but here Allen found that the homes only or mainly occupied by short-stay clients had a different approach to short stay and appeared more able to meet the needs of short-stay residents. So although short stay may be extremely beneficial from the point of view of the carer, there are reservations about its impact on elderly clients themselves as well as home management.

Vertical target efficiency Allen (1982, p.21) explores the targeting arrangements made for short-stay provision. Short-stay clients were found to be far more likely to be admitted from their own home and to be living with a son or daughter than long-stay clients. As far as reasons for admission to short stay were concerned, by far the most popular reasons were the provision of a holiday or relief for a carer or a holiday for the old person. This evidence of good targeting, however, was offset by evidence that a significant number of short-stay admissions had received no prior domiciliary support, despite protestations that 'everything' had been tried.

All six of the innovations in the short-stay group reported some targeting policy, most usually for the support of stressed relatives. These limited data point towards relatively strong emphasis on vertical target efficiency, but evidence is lacking on the extent of prior co-ordination with the domiciliary services.

Horizontal target efficiency No schemes reported uptake or outreach activity. This lack of emphasis on horizontal target efficiency (when contrasted with that evident in the case of assisted lodgings schemes) can perhaps be explained through the lack of specialist staff attached to the schemes who could engage in promotional activity. Thus Allen's examination (1982, p.115) of the pattern of referrals from social workers for short-term residential care found that more than half the social workers interviewed had referred less than ten elderly people for short-term care in the previous twelve months, with referrals concentrated among a small number of social workers. There was little knowledge within the area teams of the availability of short-term care as a resource and little attention paid to policy guidelines. The adequacy of links between these schemes and informal carers also gives rise to concern, as Allen (1982, p.160) found that over a third of carers got to know about short-term care informally. One result of the lack of knowledge about short-term care was that a high proportion of short-stay residents were having repeat stays, with the danger that the resource could silt up. Allen concluded that some of those having short-term care for the first time seemed in much greater need than those having repeat stays.

Care planning There was generally little emphasis on care planning tasks as short-stay care was often seen as a discrete service in its own right. Assessment procedures were stressed in only two reports, the most detailed specification emerging from Bury's Short Stay Home (Ferlie, 1982, p.217) where assessment starts with an intake conference and continues with a regular series of review conferences leading to discharge. This was also the only scheme to report care planning activity. However, three of the schemes did report a direct work component linked to the relief of stress on informal carers or as a means of preparing an old person for possible permanent admission. Again, the Bury scheme was the only one to provide for monitoring or a key worker system. This group of schemes typically displayed little emphasis on the processes of case management.

Cost-related criteria The schemes performed better on the signs of technical efficiency. All of course provided a short-term service and all claimed to be reducing demand for long-term Part III resources. However, only two emphasised rehabilitation as an objective, reflecting the overall acceptance of carer relief as an overriding goal. Indeed five of the six schemes explicitly mentioned relative support as an objective. The schemes were mainly financed from the SSD base budget (five reports), although there was some joint finance money (two reports), including the Bury scheme, which emphasised to an unusual degree the core tasks of case management.

Organisational process The problem context reported in most schemes (four) concentrated on service failure and inflexibility rather than more global worries. This was suggestive of a bottom-up approach although there was insufficient evidence to pursue this argument further. All had started up in the last five years and three were confined to one district, although the three others had wider coverage. Links with other services and other sections of the department were poorly developed; indeed only the Bury scheme reported any joint working. This confirms the note of service isolation already apparent.

Short-term care seems to have emerged as an incremental response to the problem of carer relief in conditions of severe pressure on Part III resources. Vertical and horizontal targeting arrangements and care planning have all been given low priority. The service seems mainly focused on carer relief rather than client rehabilitation.

Support units There were three reports received of support units from Sheffield and Derbyshire (Ferlie, 1982, pp.228-234) based on the same arguments that have underpinned the development of 'campus' models of sheltered housing. Sheffield's strategy has been outlined by Macdonald, Qureshi and Walker (1984), consisting of the replacement of conventional divisions of service into domiciliary, residential and day care sections by a more integrated and flexible resource centre model. Within such centres there will be no division of staff by function but rather a number of 'community support workers'. The Elderly Persons Support Unit (EPSU) will provide a base for staff and also community facilities and will act as a centre from which outreach activity will take place.

It is worth noting possibly contradictory objectives within the EPSU brief deriving from an attachment both to gerontological and case management arguments. On the one hand Macdonald, Qureshi and Walker (1984) emphasise the role of participation by elderly consumers in service delivery as a means of combating the negative stereotypes of passivity in old age. Thus centre workers are to be 'accountable' to local consumers. This 'extensive' objective diverges from the second 'intensive' aim of managing care for highly dependent elderly people through providing a 'full' alternative to residential care. The first objective points away from the tyranny of the case; the second reinforces it. Thus community support workers are expected to develop needs rather than service-based approaches to assessment and to construct individual care packages involving interweaving with other statutory, voluntary and informal sources of care. The EPSU programme is undergoing evaluation, although research has just started. It will be interesting to discover the results of this initiative.

In conclusion, the processes of innovation observable in this chapter are in many ways typical of change patterns within SSDs as a whole. The care system is undergoing differentiation as new services develop over time, often from a rudimentary base within the SSD. Incremental additions to service content are emphasised more than case management. The rationales for innovation vary from one context to another, with bottom-up approaches observable in some (such as assisted lodgings) but less evident in the field of day care. Processes of innovation seem service rather than agency specific.

Case Studies

Southwark Social Services Department: day centre for elderly mentally infirm people

The target group of users is seen as more demanding than those elderly people attending mainstream day centres as behaviour would be likely to warrant a much higher level of supervision. It is seen as closely linked to NHS provision and also with supporting caring families.

Target groups are tightly defined as follows: to prevent admission to, or facilitate discharge from, residential or hospital care; and to provide support and occupation for elderly mentally frail living alone or with families.

One of the most noticeable features of the centre is the involvement of health personnel. As Table 5.2 shows, all clients are jointly assessed by a psychiatrist and a social worker as well as by day centre staff. Social work support is also available for direct work with relatives. However, the orientation is still very much on a discrete form of day care: there are no reports of care planning being undertaken with

Table 5.1
Southwark SSD day centre for
elderly mentally infirm people:
case finding

Dimension	Response
Targeting (eligibility criteria)	On margin of need for residential care/frail Post-discharge care
Targeting (client subgroups)	Elderly mentally infirm Support for relatives
Uptake	No such intention/mention
Outreach	Elderly mentally infirm/elderly severely mentally infirm
Mandatory assessment	No/no mention
Preventive surveillance	No/no mention

Table 5.2
Southwark SSD day centre for
elderly mentally infirm people:
case management

Dimension	Response
Assessment (type)	General commitment
Assessment (inputs)	Social workers
	Other psychiatric staff
Care packaging (type)	No/no mention
Care packaging (scope)	No/no mention
Arranging for additional services	No/no mention
Direct work	With other informal carers
Monitoring (type)	No/no mention
Monitoring (scope)	No/no mention
Monitoring (by whom?)	No/no mention
Audit/review?	No/no details
Key worker (role)	No/no mention
Key worker (who?)	No/no mention
Post-institutional care review	No/no mention

other resources. Other case management features (monitoring, audit/review, and key worker) are similarly absent.

There are five care staff in addition to a centre head, a deputy, a visiting psychologist and sessions from adult education tutors. The 'containment' policy for those for whom rehabilitation is not possible includes supervising bathing, toileting, etc. as well as providing a meal and administering medication. There are, however, no reports of involvement by nursing staff in the care offered by the centre.

The centre attempts to rehabilitate, or at least to maintain, its clients in a number of ways (Table 5.4). Stimulation of clients is emphasised to preserve social skills, self-care and independence. Rehabilitation is a goal where the illness is functional, but the development of coping strategies for elderly mentally infirm people is also stressed. As well as providing day care, the centre goes beyond this to act as a family resource centre, so that elderly users and their families can benefit from groupwork, social events and information dissemination. There were, however, no reports of the development of localised and improvised day care facilities more characteristic of the voluntary sector. The scheme has been funded by joint finance:

Table 5.3
Southwark SSD day centre for
elderly mentally infirm people:
care provision

Dimension	Response
Personal care	General commitment
Domestic care	Preparation of meals
Night sitting	No/no mention
Out-of-hours working	No/no mention
Specialist care (eligibility criteria)	On margin of need for institutional care Post-discharge care
Specialist care (client subgroups)	Elderly mentally infirm Socially isolated Support for relatives

Table 5.4
Southwark SSD day centre for
elderly mentally infirm people:
efficiency

Dimension	Response
Short-term commitment	No/no mention
Rehabilitation	Social skills/independence EMI coping strategies Emotional support for anxiety/depression
Lower-cost mode	Shift from institutional care Support for informal carers
Support for informal carers	Day care Relatives' support group
More efficient production process	No/no mention
Source of finance	Joint finance

the capital cost is £409,000, and the annual revenue costs are estimated at £120,000.

The scheme was partially designed to relieve pressure on residential accommodation and indeed on other day centres not specifically designed for elderly mentally infirm people. The day centre opened in 1982 to cater for those in the southern part of the borough.

Table 5.5
Southwark SSD day centre for
elderly mentally infirm people:
organisational process

Dimension	Response
Problem context	Observed failure of present service
	Pressure on hospital beds
	Demographic trends
Initiating personnel	No/no mention
Pilot?	No/no mention
Duration	Less than 5 years
Coverage	One district only

The scheme does not appear to emphasise links with other agencies or sectors of the SSD with the exception of two of the staff already mentioned as assessors: the social worker, the psychiatrist, and also a visiting psychologist. There seem to be few links with domiciliary carers or sheltered housing wardens. No arrangements for evaluation were reported.

Table 5.6
Southwark SSD day centre for
elderly mentally infirm people:
joint working

Dimension	Response
Joint working (NHS staff)	Consultants
Joint working (housing department staff)	No/no details
Individual volunteers	No/no details
Voluntary organisations	No/no details
New forms of internal cross working	Day care division
	Fieldwork service division
Evaluation (by implementors)	No/no details
Evaluation (by other internal officers)	No/no details
Evaluation (by external evaluators)	No/no details

112

Conclusion This scheme represents an important contribution to day care for elderly mentally infirm people, working in collaboration with medical and social work personnel and caring relatives, extending the task of giving relief to relatives, and providing specific forms of care both for functionally and organically-based mental illnesses.

Northamptonshire SSD meals-on-wheels re-organisation

The important feature of this scheme is the emphasis placed on technical efficiency in a high-volume, mass-production, operation.

One of the problems about the pre-re-organisation service was that the patchwork system of organisation and dependence on outside suppliers had led to service dilution and the inability to expand supply with demand. To this extent the scheme is aimed at overcoming the problem of service dilution and of improving uptake (Table 5.7). The scheme does not focus on the case management process so that the next section to consider consists of the contribution made to efficiency.

The search for technical efficiency eventually led to a decision to reduce the number of outlets by installing a number of deep freeze cabinets and delivering meals in their frozen state to the client. Checks are made of clients' ability to heat their own meals. The scheme has also reduced transport costs, standardised the quality, quantity and cost of meals, given clients an element of choice and made the delivery of meals much more flexible. The scheme is base budget funded.

Table 5.7
Northamptonshire SSD
meals-on-wheels re-organisation:
case finding

Dimension	Response
Targeting (eligibility criteria)	No/no mention
Targeting (client subgroups)	No/no mention
Uptake	Intention to raise uptake, e.g. introduction of free service, creation of more accessible resources
Outreach	No/no mention
Mandatory assessment	No/no mention
Preventive surveillance	No/no mention

Table 5.8
Northamptonshire SSD
meals-on-wheels re-organisation:
efficiency

Dimension	Response
Short-term commitment	No/no mention
Rehabilitation	No/no mention
Lower-cost mode	No/no mention
Support for informal carers	No/no mention
More efficient production process	Promotion of economies of scale
Source of finance	SSD base budget

The scheme is now making a substantial contribution to changes in mainstream practice. The scheme has been retained beyond the evaluation report and covers the whole county.

Little joint working was reported except for with the WRVS (Table 5.10). In fact, the difficulty of maintaining a steady supply of volunteers was one of the motivating factors behind the re-organisation.

An evaluation was completed by the SSD research department which concluded that many of the previous problems had been solved by the re-organisation and that the new system was enabling the SSD

Table 5.9
Northamptonshire SSD
meals-on-wheels re-organisation:
organisational process

Dimension	Response
Problem context	Observed failure of present service: excessive rigidity Demographic trends
Initiating personnel	No/no mention
Pilot?	Post-pilot phase
Duration	Less than 5 years
Coverage	Authority-wide; more than one authority

Table 5.10
Northamptonshire SSD
meals-on-wheels re-organisation:
joint working

Dimension	Response
Joint working (NHS staff)	No/no details
Joint working (housing department staff)	No/no details
Individual volunteers	Tried but failed
Voluntary organisations	Local branch of Women's Royal Voluntary Service
New forms of internal cross working	No/no details
Evaluation (by implementors)	No/no details
Evaluation (by other internal officers)	SSD research and development section
Evaluation (by external evaluators)	No/no details

to supply meals in situations which would otherwise prove difficult and expensive.

Conclusion This scheme focuses on the improvement of technical efficiency in a high volume, mass market product, demonstrating the importance questions of technical efficiency have in at least some SSD-produced services.

6 Innovation in the National Health Service

Commentary

This chapter analyses 43 NHS innovations reported in Ferlie, Challis and Davies (1983) which were based in geriatric or psychogeriatric wards, the nursing or physiotherapy services or primary care settings. Detailed examples are taken from Ferlie (1982). Although the nature of the scheme varies with its base within the NHS, the historic neglect of care for elderly people and attempts to upgrade the quality of care remain common themes. The achievement of greater efficiency in the health care of elderly people is of major importance in terms of resources: elderly people occupy nearly 50 per cent of NHS hospital beds, including about 40 per cent of acute beds (Cmnd 8173, 1981).

The signs of efficiency derived reflect the twin concerns of service content and case management. Both are vital in geriatric and psychogeriatric medicine. In terms of service content, the development of rehabilitative techniques to care for elderly patients suffering from conditions such as stroke or incontinence, or at risk of falling, has been a long-standing theme of policy (Cmnd 8173, 1981) held back by the inability of geriatricians to secure beds in district general hospitals and by the traditional lack of prestige attached to geriatric nursing. As late as 1981, only about half the total nursing staff in departments of geriatric medicine were qualified (Cmnd 8173, 1981, p.54).

Case management has also featured prominently in the development of geriatric and psychogeriatric medicine given the presence of 'syndromes' of pathology including social, physical and psychiatric elements. As early as 1966, Kay, Foster and Garside (1966) pointed to the need for a geriatric service to interweave with 'lines of defence' within the community. Acute discharge policies are likely to run into obstacles if sufficient community resources are not available to support recent discharges or to act as early warning systems. Within psychogeriatrics, an emphasis on the maintenance of the demented at home also results in priority being accorded to interweaving with social services (Hemsi, 1981).

The 'bed-blocking' problem within geriatric medicine adds extra credence to the case management argument. Previous studies have found that up to a third of beds on acute medical wards can be 'blocked' by elderly patients who are no longer in need of acute medical care (McArdle, Wylie and Alexander, 1975). The development of higher turnover rates was one of the primary objectives of geriatric medicine in its attempt to shake off the 'chronic sick ward' label. Burley, Currie, Smith and Williamson (1979) report the results of a scheme of attachment to acute medical wards of geriatric consultants. They found that the mean stay was reduced and that the proportion discharged home increased, with correspondingly fewer being transferred to convalescent or geriatric wards. Among the aspects of a geriatrician's skills which they suggest could explain these changes, a number related to features of case management. They stress the importance of multidisciplinary assessment, of expertise in the mobilisation of community resources and the ability to negotiate aftercare. Improved case management and service content are as much the concern of geriatricians as they are of social workers.

Vertical target efficiency

Some twenty NHS schemes reported eligibility criteria for service, less but not significantly less than the rest of the sample (Table 6.1). The criteria most frequently adopted were that the dependency level of clients should be such as to place them at the margin of admission (ten reports) or discharge (eleven reports). A good example would be Dorset's Hospital at Home scheme for psychogeriatric patients involving extra nursing posts in order to avoid hospital admission. Three consultants reported the imposition of an age range policy (over 75 or 80) as a means of concentrating intervention on priority categories.

Health services innovations were slightly but not significantly more likely than the sample as a whole to target on client subgroups (Table 6.1). The reluctance to develop precise targeting measures may be related to the multiple pathology and haphazard selection often found

Table 6.1
Signs of efficiency improvement:
National Health Service sector
compared with other sectors

Sign	Chi square	Direction
1. Targeting (eligibility criteria)	1.47	negative
2. Targeting (client subgroups)	1.35	positive
3. Uptake	8.70***	negative
4. Outreach	0.62	positive
5. Assessment (enhanced type)	8.70***	positive
6. Assessment (multidisciplinary)	4.19**	positive
7. Care packaging	12.71***	positive
8 Service arranging	6.70***	positive
9. Direct work	2.15	positive
10 Monitoring/follow-up	2.76*	negative
11. Key worker	1.57	negative
12. Personal care	(not computed)	
13. Night sitting	(not computed)	
14 Out-of-hours working	(not computed)	
15. Short-term working	3.74*	positive
16. Rehabilitation	10.76***	positive
17 Shift from institutional care	0.16	positive
18. Support for informal carers	5.51**	positive
19. More efficient production process	1.32	negative
20. Joint finance	1.36	negative
21. Replication	(not computed)	
22. Joint working with SSDs	0.15	positive

Notes
*   p at .10
**   p at .05
***   p at .01
Source: Ferlie et al. (1984).

in admissions of elderly people so that many admitted onto geriatric wards would often also have psychiatric illnesses, and those on psychiatric wards would often display physical infirmity.

Horizontal target efficiency

It has been long established (Williamson et al., 1964) that a mass of remedial disability (urinary incontinence, depression) is not reported to doctors, nor are other disabilities such as dementia which impose risk on the patient and strain on relatives (Williamson, 1981a). Given the prospect of rapid deterioration in many of the physical diseases of old age, it becomes crucial to establish mechanisms to ensure early detection and intervention. In the psychiatric field, horizontal target efficiency seems lowest in the elderly population (Cooper and Bickel, 1984). Bergmann's (1982) report of an experimental psychogeriatric service in Newcastle concluded that it had been impossible to detect 'early' cases through primary health care channels:

> It became apparent that elderly people with early or less severe psychiatric disorders are 'invisible' to their family doctors, and even when they are in contact for medical reasons their psychiatric illness escapes detection. . . . A public health approach to the psychiatric problems of elderly people is indicated, with screening and routine assessment of vulnerable groups of elderly people as a feature.

Horizontal target efficiency is most obviously promoted through screening exercises, although they have been criticised on the basis of the small amount of pathology detected, the question of whether such pathology is remediable, the time involved and the implications for workload. In response to these objections, Williamson (1981b) suggests the development of a case-finding package of validated questions to be applied to tightly-drawn priority groups such as the 85-plus, the socially isolated and those recently discharged from hospital. Barber and Wallis' (1982) assessment of the introduction of a geriatric screening programme in a primary care setting found 78 per cent of elderly patients in the practice to have previously unrecognised or unreported problems or symptoms, but also noted a significant rise in district nurse and health visitor workload.

The health sector was significantly less likely than the rest of the sample to report measures to increase uptake (Table 6.1). Service systems which aim to intervene early and to avoid recourse to unnecessary institutionalisation may require radical changes in roles and styles of working and will be dependent on close working relationships with referring GPs. Hemsi (1982) has for instance argued that psychogeriatric services must seek to interweave far more closely with informal support networks and seek to understand an elderly person's social environment in a way which would be most difficult in a hospital-based team. Many of the innovations reported were still based on hospital beds and faced questions of which ward system to adopt and the development of links between different hospital-based services.

The health sector reported greater outreach activity than the rest of the sample, although the difference was not significant (Table 6.1). However, this was influenced by the number of incontinent laundry services in the health sector that were anxious to secure a greater number of referrals. Despite efforts by psychogeriatricians to promote more community-orientated styles of working, only three NHS schemes reported outreach activity in the care of elderly mentally infirm people.

The screening exercises reported were often undertaken at primary care level leaving open the question of links with the hospital-based services. Thus five screening exercises reported GP involvement, two health visitor and nursing input and only one a consultant input. The results of the screening exercises also varied (Ferlie, 1982), no doubt reflecting the level of resources which they had been able to attract: one discovered little remediable pathology, although another reported that, on recall, two-thirds of detected problems had been solved.

Case management

The sector performed well on this block of 'signs' (Table 6.1). Health sector schemes were significantly more likely than the rest of the sample to report an enhanced type of assessment with nearly half the health service schemes stressing 'whole person' assessments and eight reporting a policy of domiciliary assessments. Nor need the emphasis on assessment be concentrated on the period of admission to hospital care. Guy's Assessment Flats provide a 'staging post' during which assessment of the ability of clients to cope at home can take place. This confirms Isaacs' argument (1981) that comprehensive assessment represents a distinguishing aspect of geriatric medicine in addition to the more conventional diagnostic and therapeutic skills of acute medicine.

Health service schemes were significantly more likely to report multidisciplinary assessment procedures, confirming an emphasis on the assessment process. Besides consultant and nursing inputs, social workers were the group most likely to be involved (eight reports) indicating an interest in social factors and family dynamics in medical work with elderly people. Yet few reports were received of assessment procedures which involved relatives or clients or which were explicit about the range of needs considered in the assessment process. The assessment process in the Oxford Floating Beds schemes seems to reflect a wider view of assessment than is often the case in geriatric-based innovations (Ferlie, 1982). A complete medical evaluation is carried out on entry to the programme and on each subsequent admission the patient is reviewed. A medical social worker sees the patient before admission to the programme and is in continuing contact with the family and patient, and an occupational therapist continues assessment of the patient's functional competence.

The sector was significantly more likely to report care packaging and service arranging activity (Table 6.1). However, care packaging was often restricted to internal NHS resources with only three reports including SSD domiciliary care and five Part III. There seemed also to be weak links with sheltered housing (one report only) as well as voluntary and informal inputs (two reports each).

Despite the importance of the primary care sector, only three reports indicated GP involvement in a care package with activity within the primary care sector concentrated on screening exercises. Concern has been expressed about the effectiveness with which the primary care sector meets the needs of elderly people. Thompson (1981) argues that GPs may tend to underestimate the needs of their elderly patients for service and overrely on repeat prescriptions rather than active intervention. However, primary care practice, he argues, can be improved if there is access to a skilled geriatric unit which can provide good back up and co-operation. The further development of the role of liaison nurse in co-ordinating discharge and admission policies could be valuable. The report from Moorgreen Hospital's Psychogeriatric Unit outlines the role of community psychogeriatric nurses in building links with GP practices through an attachment scheme (Ferlie, 1982).

Nearly half the schemes in the NHS sector reported the provision of direct work. The proportion was somewhat higher than in the rest of the sample, although the difference was not significant (Table 6.1). Often this would be provided by firm-attached social workers, although role flexibility was also evident. Isaacs, Livingstone and Neville (1972) showed that requests for hospital admission often followed on from the breakdown in informal care networks so it is not surprising that the objectives of direct work in hospital settings would often revolve around understanding the psychodynamics which surround a request for admission (often emergency admission). For example informal carers will frequently display feelings of anxiety and stress relating to the burden they undertake but also guilt at the thought of relinquishing their caring role. A family may be internally divided regarding the acceptable level of burden or alternatively may attempt to make a scapegoat of the elderly relative. Hemsi (1981) argues that direct work can be supplemented through self-help and relatives' groups which enable family members to air and work through such feelings.

Follow-up arrangements are part of any comprehensive system of case management and especially prominent in geriatric and psychogeriatric medicine, where changes in patients' needs will have to be picked up if the necessary re-arrangements are to be made to the care package. The health sector was significantly more likely than the rest of the sample to report a monitoring or follow-up facility (Table 6.1). Nor need follow-up tail off after a short period of time. Ratna (1982) describes a psychogeriatric crisis intervention service which involved continuing domiciliary follow-up. Follow-up was most often undertaken by nurses (ten reports), although social workers and occupational therapists were also often involved (seven reports each).

Key worker systems have been commended as a means of promoting case management within the health sector, although they could be perceived as threatening the traditional co-ordinating role of the consultant. Hemsi (1981) distinguishes between treatment — which he argues to be properly the preserve of physicians — and management, where some roles (such as counselling) are less well defined as the territory of any single group. Other 'grey' areas which could indicate the need for a key worker system to facilitate management included the respective roles of day centres as against day hospitals, the choice between Part III and hospital admission and the need for relatives to have a single point of contact. Hemsi argues that either a case conference or a key worker system could be fruitfully developed in order to provide more effective case management of psychogeriatric patients. The health sector was somewhat less likely to report the adoption of a key worker system than the rest of the sample, although the difference was not significant (Table 6.1).

Case management in psychogeriatric medicine

A case management mentality is even more apparent in the psychogeriatric than in the geriatric sector, although the number of reports from psychogeriatricians (six) was too small to permit statistical analysis. Nevertheless it is instructive to examine the distinctive style which characterises the subsector. Arie and Isaacs (1978) suggest that such services will generally aim to maintain elderly people at home through taking responsibility from the first point of contact, providing initial domiciliary assessment and organising care through a multidisciplinary team which should interweave with GPs and informal carers. The characteristic ideology is community-based and role flexible, although it may be difficult to put this model into practice. Nevertheless, care of elderly mentally infirm people (especially the demented) takes place within a context where the curative assumptions of traditional acute medicine hold very badly and where there is interest in providing continuing care in the community.

As far as case finding was concerned, four of the six schemes reported in Ferlie (1982) displayed enhancements. One firm had attempted to improve liaison with GPs and another attached community psychiatric nurses to GP practices to improve the early identification of cases and in order to provide back-up for the primary health care team. A third firm used community psychiatric nurses to follow up discharged patients and also to provide an early warning system. Early identification of cases was associated with the no waiting list policy which was explicitly mentioned in two cases.

Moving on to case management, there were also attempts to enhance assessment procedures. Four schemes stressed the importance of domiciliary assessments, with another firm providing a special assessment unit. Two firms mentioned joint geriatrician and psychogeriatrician assessment procedures, and two others moved towards more collegial forms of assessment. In one scheme domiciliary assessment included a social history incorporating a list of significant informal carers with their views on management. Another scheme with an assessment ward also made provision for a joint ward round at which other professionals in addition to the consultant were represented.

There was also a substantial move towards joint working. Five of these schemes mentioned either the development of social worker, community psychiatric nurse or psychologist support, or joint work with SSD facilities, for example by taking on advice work in Part III homes. Extensive teamwork may in turn lead to a policy of greater role flexibility, as in the case of the Springfield Psychogeriatric Unit. Direct work by social workers was emphasised in one scheme with reference to carer support, counselling of the recently bereaved and of those who had attempted suicide, and work with patients discharged to Part III homes. Another scheme had appointed under joint finance a clinical psychologist to undertake inpatient group work (including reality orientation), organise a relatives' support group and liaise with social work and residential care staff over clients. Another major case management feature — the appointment of a key worker — was absent except for Springfield's prime worker system (Ferlie, 1982).

Another item considered was family support. Short-term relief admissions were mentioned in two projects, a support group in a third and one scheme provided for known key workers to be available to families, out of hours, in order to deal with crises. In a fourth scheme, community psychiatric nurses were used to build up relationships with families and to identify and support coping mechanisms. A major feature of some of these innovations therefore is the way in which attempts have been made to extend family support from the provision of specific support services (such as relief care) to building up a relationship with particular team members with the result that their needs can be more fully understood. This process may have only just begun, as few schemes involved relatives in the assessment process, but it marks an interesting development.

Follow-up work is emphasised in all these firms. This may take the form of extending the tasks of community psychiatric nurses, building links with SSD establishments to which patients may be discharged, and with SSD teams, who may also take on a responsibility for discharged patients. The report from Cambridgeshire based on a relatives' support group indicated that voluntary support was also available between meetings. Finally, Springfield has a policy of not holding routine outpatient clinics but instead relying on domiciliary visits. Springfield also placed priority on review of care policies and alteration of support in the light of changing circumstances (Ferlie, 1982).

Service content

A major question is the extent to which new nursing roles were developing. Cang (1978) argues that basic 'tending' care, applicable to many elderly patients, has acquired the status of menial work and has been relegated in importance. Although relatives often perform personal care tasks, when dependency increases tasks such as supervision of medication, lifting or changing dressings assume great importance. There was a modest development in the direction of basic nursing: eight schemes reported such provision. The best example is the Peterborough Hospital-at-home Scheme in which the new role of the patient's aide emerged. The post was defined in the following terms:

> The Patient's Aide was new, a cross between a nursing auxiliary and a home help, with a very wide job description, providing for the nursing care and monitoring of patients at home coupled with domestic and advisory support to relatives caring at home. When the posts were advertised there were 150 applicants, a large number having previously worked in hospital. They are paid the NHS rate for Auxiliary Nurses (Ferlie, 1982, p.315).

An important issue concerns the point at which basic nursing meets the new forms of personal care offered by home help services and the definition of appropriate boundaries. Management arrangements may be particularly problematic. Berkshire's home aides, whose role encompasses tasks normally carried out by different groups of NHS and SSD staff, are responsible to a joint working party, but long-term management responsibility remains unclear (Ferlie, 1982).

An attempt to develop more specialist and skilled nursing with elderly people was reported in ten schemes. In the psychogeriatric sector in particular, nursing services have traditionally been characterised by a predominance of untrained staff and have featured prominently in many inquiries (Arie and Jolley, 1982). A major recent development has been the emergence of trained community psychiatric nurses (CPNs) as a means of raising the standard of nursing in the psychiatric field given greater pressure for discharge. In some areas, CPNs are based outside the hospital and relate both to primary care and the local psychogeriatric service, although in others the CPN is a full member of the multidisciplinary team. The report from the North Manchester Psychogeriatric Unit (Ferlie, 1982, p.328) indicates that CPNs have maintained their traditional functions of administering long-term medication and acting as an early warning system, but have also moved on to counselling relatives and providing support to wardens and Part III establishments.

Cost-related criteria

Stress on cost-related criteria is evident in NHS innovations. Concern that geriatric patients should receive better access to district general hospital facilities has been balanced by fear of the resource consequences of moving to a higher unit cost mode of provision and by efforts to reduce 'bed blocking'. Cmnd 8173 argued:

> Elderly people have a right to the same standard of hospital care as is available to other age groups. And since their demands are increasing, every effort must be made to plan efficiently for their special needs. Scarce resources can be wasted if a hospital stay is unnecessarily prolonged. This can happen if facilities do not match up to needs; or if undue delays in gaining admission lead to the development of chronic disabilities, with the result that a patient's family may be less willing to resume responsibility when the need for hospital care is past (1981, p.49).

Some NHS schemes have attempted to reduce 'bed blocking' through the introduction of short-term services. Such services were reported by 24 of the NHS sector schemes, a significantly higher proportion than the sample as a whole (Table 6.1). Moreover, not all of these schemes were narrowly conceived as post-hospital discharge schemes, as relief care (five schemes) and crisis intervention (seven schemes) were also mentioned as important developments.

Rehabilitation is a second way in which bed blocking can be reduced. Thirty NHS schemes reported rehabilitative working, a significantly higher proportion than the sample as a whole (Table 6.1). The largest subcategory unsurprisingly consisted of physical rehabilitation (twelve schemes). Physical rehabilitation will be an important objective in many geriatric services, and some consultants maintain special rehabilitation wards, arguing that such wards offer better facilities and ensure that adequate staff time is made available (Pathy,

1982) for rehabilitative as well as acute work. There are of course obstacles to pursuing rehabilitative objectives. Brocklehurst and Tucker's (1980) survey of day hospitals found that staff defined physical rehabilitation as the most common reason for attendance, but also that there was a substantial number of patients staying for a longer period than implied by this objective. The next most frequently mentioned form of work was with elderly mentally infirm people, often focused on the identification of coping mechanisms for the demented through extended community nurse backup. Few NHS schemes provided social skills rehabilitation (two reports only), although the assessment flats introduced by Guy's as a means of smoothing the transition from a hospital ward to the home environment show that this objective can be pursued in a NHS setting.

Relief care for relatives has been an important feature of geriatric medicine at least since De Largy's (1957) scheme for intermittent admission. Geriatric and psychogeriatric medicine emphasises support for informal carers as a means of reducing pressure on long-term hospital beds: 25 schemes reporting informal carer support as a feature of service, a significantly higher proportion than the rest of the sample (Table 6.1). The picture described by Isaacs, Livingstone and Neville (1972) of relatives demanding hospital places for the elderly person after their own burden had become insupportable has had a pervasive effect on service style. Nor is this support seen purely in practical terms: there were reports of establishing relatives' support groups. Cambridgeshire reported the joint appointment of a clinical psychologist working with relatives and Part III staff.

On the other hand NHS schemes were less likely than the rest of the sample to pay attention to the efficiency of the production process itself, although the difference was not significant. The item most frequently mentioned in this category was the provision of training, often for new basic grade staff to improve skill levels.

Many more schemes in the sector proceeded on the basis of NHS base budget money (33 schemes) than joint finance (eleven schemes). The sector was less likely to report the use of joint finance than the rest of the sample, although the difference was not significant (Table 6.1).

Organisational process

A key question in analysing NHS schemes is the extent to which they are consultant controlled and fit a professionalised model of innovation. If autonomous professionals are in control of NHS innovations, this may make alignment with SSD innovations more difficult to achieve. In addition, a highly professionalised innovation process

126

may place little priority on the pursuit of cost-effectiveness objectives. Against this, Carboni (1982) argues that whereas in the USA collegial professionalism has emerged as the dominant form of institutional control, in the UK state mediation (through the DHSS) has always been more important. Purely professionalised processes are less likely than a loose coalition between an emerging (but still weak) segment of the medical profession and managerial patrons on which it has historically depended. Bodies such as joint care planning teams could be seen to be a recent development of continuing managerial interest in pushing forward geriatric medicine at local level. In this chapter, we are dealing with discrete schemes. The pattern of diffusion across district boundaries has been considered elsewhere (Stocking, 1985). The rate of diffusion was found to vary considerably according to the content of the scheme: reality orientation therapy appeared to diffuse at a faster rate than five-day rehabilitation wards.

The evidence from Ferlie, Challis and Davies (1983) suggests both professional and managerial interest in the process of innovation. Service development, which could be regarded as falling within the remit of a professional, was the reason most frequently cited (seventeen schemes), but other reasons more compatible with managerial priorities were also mentioned. Thus pressure on Part III (twelve schemes), pressure on hospital beds (eight schemes) and demographic trends (seven schemes) were also sometimes given as explanations for the launching of an innovation. Certainly consultants were a group often reported as the initiating personnel (eleven schemes) but other channels were also important. Thus joint NHS/SSD groups were mentioned in eleven schemes and NHS managers in nine.

The relative unimportance of short-term money in this sector has resulted in less of an emphasis on pilot schemes: only five schemes were reported to be on pilot status, a much lower proportion than in either the home help or SSD case management sectors. Similarly a higher proportion of schemes in the NHS sector reported a duration of more than five years. Taken together, these two signs indicate a lesser degree of marginality of innovations in the NHS than in the SSD sectors which may be a positive aspect of reliance on base budget money as a means of promoting innovation.

Finally, what does this information tell us about the pattern of joint working in NHS innovations? There were relatively weak links with housing departments (four schemes), voluntary organisations (three schemes) or individual volunteers (seven schemes). The strongest links were reported with two groups of SSD personnel: social workers (twenty schemes) and residential care staff (fourteen schemes). Many of the social workers will of course be attached to a consultant's team, but the number of schemes reporting links with Part III establishments is high. Nevertheless, the sector was no more likely to report joint working with SSDs than the housing and voluntary sectors (Table 6.1).

So in conclusion, NHS innovations stressed case management processes and the enhancement of nursing service content. It seemed that case management was even stronger in psychogeriatric than in geriatric settings. However, NHS innovations faced difficulty in improving horizontal target efficiency and in adopting a key worker system, indicating the continuing power of a hospital location and of consultants to restrict the move to multidisciplinary, community-based working. In terms of technical efficiency, the sector was strong on the introduction of short-term services, rehabilitation and support for informal carers. There was little use of joint finance reported by the NHS (lending credence to the argument that SSDs dominate allocation). It was also noticeable that few innovations were reported from GPs, the bulk coming from consultants or nursing services. Some GPs are said to find work with elderly people dull and unrewarding, especially single-handed doctors who lack access to team back-up (McAlpine, 1983). The pace of development in primary care for elderly people lags behind even the patchy evolution of hospital services.

Case Studies

The nature and process of innovation may vary according to the particular medical setting. Schemes based on geriatric inpatient care may vary from those launched by hospital psychogeriatric departments. Primary care-based innovations may vary again in their emphasis. The three examples chosen should illustrate differences as well as similarities in the nature of innovation in various NHS settings.

Springfield Psychogeriatric Unit

The unit works with patients over 75 suffering both from dementia and from functional disorders such as depression or anxiety. The device used to improve case finding is the provision of a quick response referral process (see Table 6.2). The service is available on a 24-hour basis with patients assessed and reviewed at home before management decisions are made. In addition, staff home telephone numbers are available to patients and their families. A medical screening is also used to detect remediable physical disorders.

An initial assessment is made at home, usually by the consultant, of the overall needs of the elderly client. Urgent admissions are dealt

Table 6.2
Springfield Psychogeriatric Unit:
case finding

Dimension	Response
Targeting (eligibility criteria)	Over 75
Targeting (client subgroups)	Elderly mentally infirm
Screening	GP-based
Uptake	No such intention/mention
Outreach	No/no mention
Referral process	Extension of scope of assessment – pre-admission
Preventive surveillance	No/no mention

with on the acute ward. A range of social work, nursing and hospital resources is available, with a community psychiatric nurse available to work with patients in their own homes. The social worker undertakes direct work with clients and informal carers. No outpatient clinics are arranged as staff go directly to patients' homes for follow-up work. Prime workers are designated but it is unclear from the present reports to what extent precise and explicit case management functions are undertaken by those so nominated.

The community psychiatric nursing service has already been mentioned. Services such as a post-discharge home help service seem less evident in psychiatric than in geriatric settings and do not appear to be present in this sample.

Short-term acute beds are available for relief admissions or crisis intervention (Table 6.5). For the many patients exhibiting signs of dementia, alleviation is a more realistic objective than rehabilitation. The move away from chronic institutional care is augmented by the use of day- and short-term care to relieve relatives, although little use is reported of more localised voluntary resources. The unit is NHS base budget financed.

The unit is a new one, set up in 1979 in order to offer a specific and specialised service for elderly people, especially those suffering from dementia. Although the unit has an attached social worker, links with other parts of the SSD and with the housing department responsible for sheltered housing could be developed further. Emphasis is placed on developing better relations with GPs.

Table 6.3
Springfield Psychogeriatric Unit:
case management

Dimension	Response
Assessment (type)	Focus on problems/strengths rather than eligibility for service
	Assessment at home
Assessment (inputs)	Consultant psychogeriatricians
No waiting list for admission	Yes
Treatment/care packaging	SSD fieldwork services
	Psychiatric community nurses
	NHS day hospitals
	NHS acute psychogeriatric beds
	Rehabilitative psychogeriatric beds
	NHS continuing care psychogeriatric beds
Arranging for additional services	No/no mention
Direct work (by whom?)	Social worker
Direct work (role)	With client/patient
	With other informal carers
Follow-up (by whom?)	Health visitors
Follow-up (role)	Home nursing care
	Domiciliary outpatient visits
	Work with Part III residents
Key worker (role)	Co-ordination
Key worker (who?)	Social workers/health visitors
	Nurses/nursing officers
	Consultant geriatricians

Table 6.4
Springfield Psychogeriatric Unit:
care provision

Dimension	Response
Skilled nursing care	General commitment
Basic nursing care	No/no mention
Other care	No/no mention
Specialist care (eligibility criteria)	No/no mention
Specialist care (client subgroups)	Elderly mentally infirm

Table 6.5
Springfield Psychogeriatric Unit:
efficiency

Dimension	Response
Short-term/acute service available	Relief care
	Crisis work
	Acute beds
Rehabilitation	EMI coping strategies
Lower-cost mode	Shift from institutional care
	Support for informal carers
Support for informal carers	Day care
	Relief residential care
	Direct work/bereavement therapy
More efficient production process	No/no mention
Source of finance	Internal NHS base budget

Table 6.6
Springfield Psychogeriatric Unit:
organisational process

Dimension	Response
Problem context	Observed failure of present service
Initiating personnel	Consultant psychogeriatricians
	NHS management
Pilot?	No/no mention
Duration	Less than 5 years
Joint working (SSD staff)	Social workers
	Residential care staff
Joint working (housing department staff)	No/no details
Individual volunteers	No/no details
Voluntary organisations	No/no details
New forms of internal NHS joint working	GPs
	Consultant psychogeriatricians
Evaluation (by implementors)	No/no details
Evaluation (by other internal officers)	No/no details
Evaluation (by external evaluators)	No/no details

The admission policy in the Leeds unit provides for an age-related service embracing the over 85s and including the over 75s when resources permit. Although as the unit is a hospital-based service referrals are generated through GPs rather than directly, emphasis can fruitfully be placed on encouraging referrals by establishing health visitors for liaison tasks and ensuring that the consultant is generally available to speak to enquiring GPs (Table 6.7). As geriatrics units return more elderly people to the community and thus hand over responsibility to primary health care teams, facilities for urgent re-admission, day hospital care and outpatient review are crucial.

The distinctive feature in the case management process is the adoption of a single ward system rather than the traditional pattern of acute, rehabilitation and long-stay wards. It is thought that as a result of this policy turnover increases and waiting lists are diminished with the result that more acute admissions can be accepted. Other dimensions of case management are not so prominent except for the follow-up role undertaken by health visitors. There is little mention of closer operational links with social services staff or of the key worker system noticeable in some psychiatric settings.

Stress is laid on supporting members of the primary health care team in coping with patients discharged home by making hospital facilities more readily available. No mention was made of an enhanced role for community nurses or of social workers in the follow-up phase.

The single ward system claims a number of advantages as far as service efficiency is concerned. Vacancies appearing in the previous

Table 6.7
St James' Single Geriatric Ward:
case finding

Dimension	Response
Targeting (eligibility criteria)	Over 75
Targeting (client subgroups)	No/no mention
Screening	No/no mention
Uptake	No such intention/mention
Outreach	No/no mention
Referral process	More direct access to services by GPs
Preventive surveillance	No/no mention

Table 6.8
St James' Single Geriatric Ward:
case management

Dimension	Response
Assessment (type)	Assessment in hospital
Assessment (inputs)	Consultant geriatricians
No waiting list for admission	Yes
Treatment/care packaging	No/no mention
Arranging for additional services	No/no mention
Direct work (by whom?)	No/no details
Direct work (role)	No/no details
Follow-up (by whom?)	Community psychiatric nurses
Follow-up (role)	General commitment
Key worker (role)	No/no mention
Key worker (whom?)	No/no mention

Table 6.9
St James' Single Geriatric Ward:
care provision

Dimension	Response
Skilled nursing care	General commitment
Basic nursing care	No/no mention
Other care	No/no mention
Specialist care (eligibility criteria)	Over 75
Specialist care (client subgroups)	No/no mention

'long-stay' area have been filled by selected rehabilitation patients, holiday and rotating admissions (Table 6.10). The provision of relief care in order to relieve relatives is thus seen as one way of moving away from traditional conceptions of long-term care. However, little use was made of voluntary or local resources in supporting informal carers.

The re-organisation was prompted by a growing concern of the consultant that traditional services were too inflexible and lead to long

Table 6.10
St James' Single Geriatric Ward:
efficiency

Dimension	Response
Short-term/acute service available	Relief care
	Acute beds
Rehabilitation	Physical rehabilitation
Lower-cost mode	Shift from institutional care
	Support for informal carers
Support for informal carers	Relief residential care
More efficient production process	No/no mention
Source of finance	Internal NHS base budget

delays and waiting lists. The unit's policy is to emphasise links with other health professionals in the primary health care setting (Table 6.11). The nature of relationships with other hospital firms and community-based resources such as Part III and sheltered housing facilities is not clear in the reports received.

Peterborough Hospital-at-home Scheme

The Peterborough Hospital-at-home Scheme is designed to cater for patients who would normally be cared for in hospital in their home surroundings. Its two most notable organisational features lie in the concept of patients' aides and an enhanced role for the GP.

As Table 6.12 indicates, the scheme includes the condition that if it had not been for the scheme the patient would have to be in hospital. The scheme is not targeted on any of the subgroups listed in the coding sheet, but does manage the care of the dying. Measures are not taken to increase uptake or outreach as a closed referral policy is in operation, controlled by medical personnel, mostly by the GP but also by consultants. The main contribution to improved case finding lies in the fact that GPs can make direct referral rather than have to go through hospital personnel.

The initial assessment is of course based at home. Needs can also be met by the social worker, physiotherapist and occupational therapist attached to the scheme. Clinical management is undertaken where necessary by the GP. There are thus a variety of inputs available, some across the usual organisational boundaries (Table 6.13). An

Table 6.11
St James' Single Geriatric Ward:
organisational process

Dimension	Response
Problem context	Observed failure of present service: excessive rigidity Pressure on hospital beds
Initiating personnel	Consultant geriatricians
Pilot?	No/no mention
Duration	No details
Joint working (SSD staff)	No/no details
Joint working (housing department staff)	No/no details
Individual volunteers	No/no details
Voluntary organisations	No/no details
New forms of internal NHS joint working	GPs Consultant geriatricians Community nurses
Evaluation (by implementors)	No/no details
Evaluation (by other internal officers)	No/no details
Evaluation (by external evaluators)	No/no details

Table 6.12
Peterborough Hospital-at-home Scheme:
case finding

Dimension	Response
Targeting (eligibility criteria)	On margin of admission to institutional care
Targeting (client subgroups)	Support for relatives
Screening	No/no mention
Uptake	No such intention/mention
Outreach	No/no mention
Referral process	More direct access to services by GPs
Preventive surveillance	No/no mention

Table 6.13
Peterborough Hospital-at-home Scheme:
case management

Dimension	Response
Assessment (type)	Focus on problems/strengths rather than eligibility for service
	Assessment at home
Assessment (inputs)	Social workers/health visitors
	Nursing staff/officers
	GPs
	Client
	Client's significant others/informal carers
No waiting list for admission	No/no mention
Treatment/care packaging	SSD fieldwork services
	District nurses
	OTs/physiotherapist
	GPs
Arranging for additional services	Innovation in formal procedure: SSD and NHS services
Direct work (by whom?)	Community nurses
Direct work (role)	General commitment
Follow-up (by whom?)	No/no details
Follow-up (role)	No/no details
Key worker (role)	No/no mention
Key worker (who?)	No/no mention

unusual feature of the assessment process is that for the service to be offered, the hospital-at-home nurses and social worker, the patient's relatives, the patient and the GP all have to want domiciliary care more than admission to hospital. One point relates to the failure of the first phase of the scheme in which a 'free floating' project team found the generation of referrals difficult. The administration has now been transferred to the offices of the district community nursing service, with the day-to-day running of the scheme directed by a senior nursing officer.

As Table 6.13 indicates, case management features are not emphasised. A social worker is able to undertake direct work; however, the tasks involved are not specified in present reports. There is in addition no key worker provision, at least in the reports received.

This is one of the few schemes to distinguish explicitly between skilled and basic nursing tasks, and to provide both kinds of staff. SRNs are available out of normal hours but this is supplemented by the new post of patient's aide, a cross between a nursing auxiliary and a home help, with a wide job description including domestic care tasks (Table 6.14). In many cases care is given to stroke patients. The scheme thus manages to offer a wide variety of tasks at different levels of nursing skill.

The scheme takes on patients who can be rehabilitated as well as chronic or terminal cases: about 25 per cent of the patients have been discharged. The scheme has made a major contribution to more efficient care by reducing the need for hospital places, by offering relatives domiciliary as well as social work support, and by introducing new basic grades of staff to undertake specific tasks (Table 6.15). There was, however, no reported involvement of volunteers or provision of SSD services such as domiciliary care in the scheme. Initial finance for a three years' pilot project came from the Sainsbury Family Trust in order to mount a replication of the 'Santé Service Bayonne' scheme in France. The AHA agreed to continue this pilot scheme after three years if agreed criteria of success were fulfilled and in fact such money was subsequently allocated.

Table 6.16 shows that the scheme aimed at relieving pressure on hospital beds and at enabling patients willing to be cared for at home to have this option. The idea arose from the study undertaken by the Peterborough district management team of the Santé Service Bayonne. The scheme was conceived as a pilot in one specific area but has moved on to mainstream programme status. The scheme has led to a closer working relationship between GPs, nurses and a social worker, but volunteers have not been included in the management of

Table 6.14
Peterborough Hospital-at-home Scheme:
care provision

Dimension	Response
Skilled nursing care	Out-of-hours care
Basic nursing care	Toileting
	Bathing
	Out-of-hours care
Other care	Preparation of meals
	Cleaning
Specialist care (eligibility criteria)	On margin of need for institutional care
Specialist care (client subgroups)	Stroke patients
	Support for relatives

the scheme. A thorough evaluation was built into the pilot scheme which elucidated consumer and practitioner ratings of the success of the scheme as well as complex cost comparisons which indicated that hospital-at-home costs per day were lower than in an acute hospital, but the length of care was longer.

Table 6.15
Peterborough Hospital-at-home Scheme:
efficiency

Dimension	Response
Short-term/acute service available	No/no mention
Rehabilitation	General commitment
Lower-cost mode	Shift from institutional care
	Support for informal carers
	Use of lower-cost staff
Support for informal carers	Domiciliary care
	Direct work/bereavement therapy
More efficient production process	New forms of beds
Source of finance	Private (trust)
	Internal NHS base budget

Table 6.16
Peterborough Hospital-at-home Scheme:
organisational process

Dimension	Response
Problem context	Observed failure of present service: disregard of client preferences
	Pressure on hospital beds
Initiating personnel	NHS management
Pilot?	Post-pilot phase
Duration	Less than 5 years
Joint working (SSD staff)	Social workers
Joint working (housing department staff)	No/no details
Individual volunteers	No/no details
Voluntary organisations	No/no details
New forms of internal NHS joint working	GPs
	District nurses
Evaluation (by implementors)	No/no details
Evaluation (by other internal officers)	Steering party
Evaluation (by external evaluators)	No/no details

138

7 Innovation in Housing Services

Commentary

Information was available on 31 housing-based innovations (Ferlie, Challis and Davies, 1983), mainly very sheltered housing schemes but including also a few reports of group homes and of core units. Case study information is also taken from Ferlie (1982). Before moving on to analyse these reports, the chapter outlines how housing departments have gradually accepted a function of providing special age-related provision for elderly people and of the main choices in service delivery which have been opened up.

The United Kingdom pioneered the development of sheltered housing, developing the policy some twenty years in advance of other western countries. However, the initiative in service development has often been bottom up and hence *ad hoc* in nature. Heumann and Boldy (1982, p.78) argue that national sheltered housing policies have picked up on accepted local 'good practice', that national controls have been narrowly focused on capital expenditure and that performance criteria have often been left to the local sponsor. The result has been a profusion of important variants on a common theme.

Housing-based innovations exhibit alternative housing or care rationales. The housing rationale recognises that elderly people tend to live in poorer quality housing: they are more likely to live in older property, more likely to be located within the disadvantaged private rented sector, and if they are owner occupiers, they are often unable to discharge the financial or physical burdens of upkeep (Butler, Oldman and Grieve, 1983). The care rationale argues that such housing need could be met by lower cost 'staying put' alternatives, such as home improvements, and that sheltered housing should be reserved for elderly people of higher dependency. One danger is that such a continuum of care models could result in a conveyor-belt approach with elderly clients being forced to move from one site to another to adapt to increasing levels of dependency.

The basic sheltered housing programme has now developed into a major resource. The first sheltered housing innovation is credited to Sturminster Newton Rural District Council in 1948, and early development was concentrated in the West Country. The development of liaison between local housing and welfare departments was facilitated by the 1948 Local Government Act which empowered county councils to make contributions towards the expenses of district councils. In practice this was one means of subsidising the payment of wardens' salaries. A 1961 joint circular (Ministry of Housing and Local Government and Ministry of Health, 1961) urged further co-operation between the various services for elderly people, defined the role of the warden in terms of surveillance and domestic chores, and urged joint selection of tenants to achieve a 'balanced' community which would ensure that pressure on the warden did not become excessive. The circular stated:

> Where there is a warden and particularly where the County Council have contributed to the cost, there has been a tendency to choose the tenants from among the most infirm old people. The result is that no one is fit enough to give much help to anyone else, and there is then greater pressure on the warden and a heavier demand for help from outside.

Note the stress on the lay warden role, the fear of excessive dependency and the assumption that the service would develop as a housing service for low-income elderly. Subsidy arrangements linked local welfare and housing departments to an unusual degree, but conflict over allocation policy was already evident. Although the development of sheltered housing was boosted by Townsend's (1962) influential critique of residential care which argued for an alternative policy of expansion of sheltered housing provision, this position was criticised, especially by housing department personnel (Bytheway and James, 1978) who argued that there was a danger that sheltered housing would become too much like Part III.

The different housing and care rationales lead to alternative approaches to the management of the sheltered housing stock. In

140

housing department terms, sheltered housing is often seen as a part of the mainstream housing stock which enables the authority to reduce underoccupancy and redeploy family accommodation. Thus areas with a large proportion of public housing provision also tend to have a relatively generous level of sheltered housing (Butler, Oldman and Grieve, 1983, p.67). In SSD terms, sheltered housing is seen as an alternative to increasingly pressurised residential accommodation which can, however, only cater for elderly people at higher dependency levels through extra care inputs.

This confusion about the degree to which sheltered housing should be seen in housing support or care support terms became more serious as the programme expanded. By 1963 only about 36,000 old people were thought to be living in sheltered housing, but this figure rose to an estimated 300,000 in 1976 and 400,000 in 1980 (Goldberg and Connelly, 1982, p.190). As the programme grew in size so did the need for clearer guidelines. A 1969 Circular (Ministry of Housing and Local Government, 1969) defined two types of accommodation: Category 1 would consist of self-contained private units, with or without community facilities, while Category 2 would house the less active elderly with greater emphasis on communal living. Both categories would be warden supported and have an intercom or alarm bell system. During the 1970s local experiments moved beyond this in response to increased dependency and greater demands on wardens, although there was no official updating of central government guidelines. There was also a problem that elderly people who became more frail could be expected to move again, out of conventional (especially Category 1) sheltered housing to residential care, despite the negative experiences often associated with relocation (Heumann and Boldy, 1982, p.121). In particular, a new emphasis was placed on 'linked schemes' which linked sheltered housing with a residential home and so called Category 2 provision where residents have access to on-site meals and home help support.

These new services emerged as the sheltered housing population aged and became more dependent. Heumann and Boldy (1982) provide evidence from Devon to show that between 1973 and 1977 the tenant population within sheltered housing aged and the proportion living alone increased, as did the proportion receiving statutory help. Other criticisms of the conventional sheltered housing programme have focused on a poor level of social interaction. Rosow (1967), writing in an American context, argued that the incidence of neighbouring for elderly people was higher in age-related housing. Age segregation was seen as a positive measure against loneliness and social isolation. British work has questioned this assumption. Fennell's study (1977) of the pattern of social interaction in grouped housing in Newcastle led him to reject the hypothesis that age dense housing facilitated interaction. Lipman's study (1967) of the effects of siting old people's homes near community facilities found that this did not lead to greater interaction. Criticisms of the alleged isolation engendered by some sheltered housing schemes have in turn contributed to the 'staying put' argument (Wheeler, 1982), an alternative made more feasible by the development of dispersable alarms.

Fears of the increased dependency of tenants within sheltered housing also led to the introduction of very sheltered housing or Part II schemes, in which housing support was linked up with social support. However, the co-operation between housing and social service departments (coterminous in London boroughs and metropolitan districts but not in the shire counties) crucial to such schemes had been eroded by the 1973 Housing Act which made SSD financial support to housing authorities unnecessary. Withdrawal has been slow but steady. Butler, Oldman and Grieve argue that this Act 'precipitated a breakdown' (1983, p.59) in the pattern of grants, and also the level of co-operation. The emergence of joint finance as an alternative source of subsidy may have had compensatory positive effects in stimulating liaison.

Joint finance has been especially important in funding the very sheltered housing which offers an alternative to frail elderly people which does not involve a 'conveyor-belt' move on to Part III as dependency increases, and in which realistic arrangements can be made for support which do not place unreasonable demands on lay wardens. Warwickshire SSD's (1980) pioneering efforts have been dependent on joint working between the housing and social services authorities. In the initial design of the scheme (Warwickshire SSD, 1975) it was found that up to 40 per cent of Part III admissions could have been avoided if alternatives had been available. Conventional sheltered housing had been unable to offer a true alternative because of the poor working conditions of the warden and the tenants' need to manage stairs. A joint decision was then made between the county and the district authorities that no more conventional sheltered housing should be developed and that future investment should be concentrated in very sheltered housing.

However, there have been a number of criticisms of the very sheltered housing movement. First, Tunney (1981) has drawn attention to the lack of definition. Does the term include extra facilities (such as higher staffing levels, communal dining rooms, special bathrooms and a nursing bay) or extra services (meals-on-wheels and home help)? The critique by Butler, Oldman and Grieve (1983) of very sheltered housing emphasises that the creation of an extensive very sheltered housing programme as a first point of entry exacerbates the problem of 'over attraction' of service to tenants as compared with elderly people in the community of equal dependency. In addition very sheltered housing may imply the loss of tenancy rights valued by elderly clients. Thus the Kinloss Court scheme provides for a pledge by the NHS and SSD to accept a tenant if the warden and others feel that the tenant has become too dependent (Ferlie, 1982).

Babbage (1981) outlines an alternative approach which has been developed in Hammersmith and Fulham. It was seen as questionable whether the housing service could manage specialist facilities such as very sheltered housing, in the light of criticism that it could not even discharge its basic repair and maintenance functions well. Second, there was a danger of a financially-based distortion of provision, given that councils were likely to promote such schemes in order to gain Department of the Environment approval and hence provide the basis for at least a residual new build programme. An alternative strategy was to spread tenants who needed additional care (estimated at 2 per cent of the elderly tenant population) throughout existing sheltered housing schemes, creating the space to develop a sheltering at home programme and a major grants programme aimed at maintaining elderly people in their own (upgraded) accommodation. It is for this reason that some schemes have moved towards 'sheltering at home' (Tinker, 1980) by making sheltered housing communal facilities available to elderly people in the vicinity, or by using good neighbour, peripatetic warden or dispersed alarm systems. There are, however, reservations about the reliability of some of the systems and their failure to address the social needs of isolated elderly. The viability of this model is also sensitive to the estimate of the percentage of elderly tenants who require extra care. Were this to rise, the viability of the approach would be threatened.

Vertical target efficiency

A distinction can be drawn between extensive and intensive forms of housing provision which parallel concerns of horizontal and vertical target efficiency respectively. Intensive provision is likely to provide for a small number of more dependent clients; extensive provision for a larger number of less dependent clients. The focusing of resources on very sheltered housing schemes exemplifies this intensive service orientation. A major worry has been the inability to specify clearly the level of tenant dependency for which the service should be catering. Tenants include those of slight and severe dependency as well as of moderate dependency for whom sheltered housing really would represent a halfway house between home and institutional care (D. Plank, 1977). In addition tenants in sheltered housing may well 'attract' services to a much greater degree than elderly people of equal dependency living at home, given greater visibility to key referral points such as wardens. Butler, Oldman and Wright (1979) found that of the 600 tenants studied, 16–17 per cent were receiving meals on wheels and 30 per cent home help, compared with 2.6 per cent and 8.9 per cent of elderly people living at home (Hunt, 1978).

Housing schemes were likely to report targeting by eligibility criteria in almost exactly the same proportion as the rest of the sample with seventeen schemes declaring that they targeted on those at the margin of admission for institutional care (Table 7.1). Although housing conditions remain a powerful determinant of admission to mainstream sheltered housing programmes — given the finding of Butler, Oldman and Wright (1979) that 25 per cent of tenants had previously had no

Table 7.1
Signs of efficiency improvement:
housing sector compared with other sectors

Sign	Chi square	Direction
1. Targeting (eligibility criteria)	0.15	positive
2. Targeting (client subgroups)	3.11*	negative
3. Uptake	6.14**	positive
4 Outreach	3.98**	negative
5. Assessment (enhanced type)	8.07***	negative
6. Assessment (multidisciplinary)	0.25	negative
7. Care packaging	10.35***	negative
8. Service arranging	1.35	negative
9. Direct work	7.47***	negative
10. Monitoring/follow-up	0.09	negative
11. Key worker	0.34	negative
12. Personal care	0.04	negative
13. Night sitting	(not computed)	
14. Out-of-hours working	0.29	negative
15. Short-term working	15.89***	negative
16. Rehabilitation	28.45***	negative
17. Shift from institutional care	1.00	positive
18. Support for informal carers	12.50***	negative
19. More efficient production process	0.44	negative
20 Joint finance	0.04	positive
21. Replication	3.58*	negative
22 Joint working with NHS	0.60	positive

Notes
*   p at .10
**   p at .05
***   p at .01
Source: Ferlie et al. (1984).

144

running water, 22 per cent no bathroom and 23 per cent no inside toilet (compared with Hunt's figures for the elderly population as a whole of 8 per cent, 11 per cent and 12 per cent) — housing needs are less important in the allocation of very sheltered housing tenancies. Even within the mainstream sheltered housing programme, Butler, Oldman and Grieve (1983) suggest that dependency may be becoming a more important predictor of admission over time. Whereas 69 per cent of those moving to sheltered housing in the study reported doing so for 'health' reasons, the figure for those moving more than eight years before had been only 41 per cent.

As far as targeting on client groups is concerned, the housing sector was significantly less likely to report such targeting than the rest of the sample (Table 7.1). Twelve housing based schemes reported some such targeting, usually on the physically handicapped. Only two schemes reported targeting on the socially isolated elderly, indicating that a Rosow-style social model of allocation has not been widely adopted. Few schemes (three) explicitly stated that post-discharge cases from hospital or residential care would be accepted.

There is no evidence that the degree of vertical target efficiency is significantly higher than the rest of the sample, as might be expected from such a capital intensive resource. However, compared with mainstream sheltered housing, innovatory provision follows a 'care' rather than 'housing' targeting strategy, aimed at providing an additional entry point in sheltered housing for the frail, rather than providing good quality housing and social support for a 'mix' of tenants.

Horizontal target efficiency

The advocates of extensive provision argue that it is unfair that sheltered housing residents should receive more in terms of services than equally dependent elderly people in the community (Heumann and Boldy, 1982). The traditional lack of emphasis on case-finding activity further demonstrates this intensive rather than extensive orientation.

However, the emergence of dispersed alarm systems has enabled the basic benefits of sheltered housing (alarm cover, warden support and enhanced social facilities) to be taken to elderly people in their own homes. Dispersed alarm systems will themselves have to tackle several questions: will the alarm system be appropriately used in reporting emergencies? How is the central call-in facility to be manned? How technically reliable is the system?

Eighteen schemes reported uptake activity, a significantly higher proportion than the rest of the sample (Table 7.1). Often uptake activity was based on the introduction of a mobile warden service and remote alarm facility which enabled the warden service to be offered to those in their own home. The Sheltering at Home project run by Hammersmith on Inner Areas Programme money provides not only a remote warden service but also social facilities in a local community centre (Ferlie, 1982). However, very little outreach activity was undertaken (Table 7.1).

Few reports were received of the emergence of a 'campus' model of housing-based care in the UK context in which residential facilities are linked in with a wider network of community-based services within a resource centre concept. Philadelphia Geriatric Center's Community Housing Programme (Brody, 1978), for example, enables tenants (selected mainly on social rather than dependency grounds) to have access to an emergency communications system, social work support, the Centre's social events and a 'buy-in' facility for domestic care and home-delivered frozen main meals. Other American experiments combine housing with limited support, intermediate and residential care, and skilled or long-term nursing on one site (Hearnden, 1983). Four reports only were received (Ferlie, 1982) of the development of core or support projects. For example, the Polegate Project provides for the linked use of Part III beds, a special intensive care unit with nursing support, sheltered housing and community outreach operating from two sites.

Other devices to increase horizontal target efficiency include the provision of community-based warden and alarm systems (often in improvised settings such as tower blocks), the use of day care in sheltered housing as an outreach measure and in one case the construction of a care team which took on aids and adaptations work for the whole of the elderly population. In another case, a community warden scheme was also used to increase the take-up rate of improvement grants.

Case management

The potentially conflicting housing and care objectives of the sheltered housing programme have already been noted. The 1977 Green Paper on Housing (Cmnd 6951) drew attention to the implications of this:

> The implementation of Government policy on the care of elderly people depends upon local housing authorities being fully involved with health and social service authorities in establishing effective methods of assessing need, planning provision, providing facilities and allocating resources. There is considerable scope for fuller co-operation in planning service developments in the three fields and for co-ordination of administrative policies — for example admission and discharge procedures in hospital and residential homes, and tenancy allocation procedures for housing (para. 12.41).

146

As the allocation process is vital to any such interagency co-operation, evidence relating to disagreements between housing and SSD staff in allocation policy is disturbing. Bytheway and James (1978) conducted research into the attitudes of housing and SSD officers to the allocation of sheltered housing tenancies, finding conflicting professional ideologies between the two groups of staff which presented substantial barriers to effective joint working. In Butler, Oldman and Grieve's study (1983) of twelve areas, the housing department had control of allocations in most areas and in only one authority was the SSD actively involved in the assessment of applicants for sheltered housing. The more usual system was one of nominations and recommendations of either a formal or informal nature, with (paradoxically) tensions between the two departments increasing when formal liaison machinery was established. The community physician could exert a greater influence on the allocation of sheltered housing than social workers, as the concept of medical rather than social need appeared more salient to housing department allocators. An important side effect of a continuing housing orientation to the allocation of tenancies was indirect bias against elderly owner occupiers, due to the operation of a points system which effectively excluded a large group of elderly people from the service. This paints a depressing picture for those who argue that sheltered housing could represent an important new point on a continuum of care. Against this it was also apparent (Butler, Oldman and Grieve, 1983, p.96) that the internal organisation of a housing department affects the management style of sheltered housing. In some authorities powerful specialist subsections concerned with sheltered housing have emerged which control a large proportion of the capital budget. These specialist subsections in turn take on something of a social services ideology without the direct involvement of the SSD. The North Hertfordshire Sheltered Housing Support Care Team (Ferlie, 1982, p.386) represents a good example of this line of development.

However, the move to very sheltered housing with more explicit caring roles potentially increases SSD input into the assessment process. The first question is the depth of the assessment process. Only three housing-based schemes reported an enhanced type of assessment, a significantly lower proportion than the rest of the sample (Table 7.1). It is noteworthy that a major long-term resource should be allocated in so cavalier a fashion.

The second question is that of joint assessment. Twelve housing schemes reported the operation of a multidisciplinary procedure (usually incorporating health, SSD and housing department representatives): a lower proportion than the rest of the sample, although this difference was not significant. Such panels display a wide variety of criteria for admission. Salford's Eccles scheme specifies that applications can be considered from those in housing need or from those who could be discharged from Part III homes or residential care to a supported environment (Ferlie, 1982). Wide-ranging criteria for tenancy allocation may re-open debates about the role of sheltered housing as well as providing a more rounded approach to allocation.

The same case management arguments apply to care packaging functions, which assume increased importance in very sheltered housing settings where care services are provided. This in turn requires good liaison between housing and social services at operational as well as at planning level. However, care planning was explicitly reported in only three housing-based schemes, mostly in those developments which had moved towards the role of a service campus or resource centre. Reported care packaging was significantly less in the housing sector than in the rest of the sample (Table 7.1). No care planning was reported in most of the very sheltered housing schemes, with support services such as home or community nursing often provided by separate line management hierarchies with no arrangements for client level co-ordination.

Explicit service arranging capability was reported in two schemes only. The amount of direct work support provided was significantly less in the housing sector than the rest of the sample (Table 7.1). Social work counselling was explicitly mentioned in only four schemes, mostly group homes which might require initial social work support in order to establish a group identity. The Polegate project was one of the few very sheltered housing schemes to report direct work functions which included individual counselling, group work and relatives' support groups (Ferlie, 1982).

There were few reports (six) of procedures designed to ensure that need was reviewed and re-assessed through a monitoring system (Table 7.1), although the housing sector was broadly in line with the rest of the sample. In three cases assessment took place in an assessment or rehabilitation unit attached to a sheltered housing site. In one project based on a campus model, the management team took on the regular re-assessment of client needs and of the allocation of services over which they had direct control. In the other two projects, regular reviews of home help provision were undertaken. In general, however, there was little emphasis on re-examining provision with tenancies allocated either for life or until increased dependency forced admission to institutional care. Of course one of the main advantages to the consumer of sheltered housing is precisely the security conferred by the tenancy.

In only three schemes was a key worker system used to pull together services, although this proportion was in line with the rest of the sample (Table 7.1). The evidence indicates that a relatively low priority is accorded to case management functions despite the need to integrate housing and SSD support within very sheltered housing innovations.

Service content

If developments in care planning are not a priority, emphasis might instead be placed on changing service content with moves to service rich sites where support can be expected to be more flexible and varied. Twenty-four schemes reported domestic care support, five reported an out-of-hours service and several others reported a group basis for working with a group of home helps being attached to a specific site. Moreover, eleven schemes reported personal care support. The proportion reporting personal care and out-of-hours working was almost exactly the same as in the rest of the sample, indicating that further moves could be made to a more flexible and varied service. In addition very few housing-based schemes indeed reported any form of nursing cover.

An important service content issue relates to the role of the wardens, which has emerged as a major anomaly: they are crucial to the support system, yet lack professional status. In Fox's study (1981), wardens felt unable to deal on terms of equality with other workers (a quarter of wardens were classified as manual workers) and felt that they received little help from other support services. The position of the warden has become increasingly difficult as demands have increased both in volume and complexity, yet job descriptions often remain vague, pay rates low and training facilities rudimentary. Certainly many wardens are now performing considerably more than their original role of 'good neighbours', undertaking essentially super-visory tasks (Age Concern, 1972). Butler, Oldman and Grieve (1983) found in their study that 48 per cent of wardens had supervised medication within the last week, 28 per cent had cooked a meal for the tenants, and 34 per cent helped with bathing or dressing. Clearly roles are being renegotiated, often with resistance from wardens, who are facing increasing workloads. Heumann and Boldy (1982, p.139) found that between 1973 and 1977 there was roughly a 50 per cent increase in the working week of a sample group of wardens. Extra duties were evident in schemes designed for more dependent elderly: Category 2 wardens were found to spend more time on completing home help tasks and to use more meal planning skills.

In terms of the expansion of the role of the warden, the main developments reported are the growth of extended coverage on a seven-day or 24-hour basis (nine schemes), the appointment of mobile

149

or home wardens (five schemes) and a drift towards higher staffing ratios, although this was reflected more in support staff than in the appointment of more wardens. Few reports were received of changing the job descriptions of wardens in order to reflect increased responsibilities — the Polegate Project proving an exception to this providing a job description which incorporates a larger care element.

However, developments in other support services were mentioned more frequently. Ten schemes (30 per cent) mentioned improved design features. A good example comes from Harlow in which 10 per cent at least of the dwellings are to be designed to full wheelchair standards and a large proportion are to have such features as sliding doors, low-level fitments and bath and kitchen aids (Ferlie, 1982). In these cases, enhanced design is being used to create an 'artificial' environment which stimulates independent living.

Cost-related criteria

The housing sector performed poorly on key cost-related criteria. It was significantly less likely than the rest of the sector to report short-term working (Table 7.1). There were only three reports of a short-term or acute service being available, one in a 'linked' short-term special intensive care unit, which was also the only mention made of attempts to rehabilitate tenants should they become increasingly frail. There are significantly fewer reports of rehabilitative activity in the sector than in the rest of the sample (Table 7.1).

On the other hand, the sector was rather more likely than the rest of the sample to report a shift from institutional care, although the difference was not significant (Table 7.1). Warwickshire's costing of the very sheltered housing programme argued that even at this intensive level of provision the cost to the SSD of each very sheltered unit was £76 per week less than a Part III place, whereas the cost to the housing department was seen as similar to a conventional housing scheme (Warwickshire SSD, 1980). Nearly all the reports in Ferlie, Challis and Davies (1983) claimed to be acting as an alternative to conventional Part III provision, but there were few such clear and detailed costings. Neither was a sheltered housing service seen as a means of offering additional support to stressed relatives in the manner clearly noticeable in many domiciliary care schemes. The sector was significantly less likely to offer support to informal carers than the rest of the sample (Table 7.1).

A major drawback of sheltered housing is the large capital cost involved in providing for a relatively small number of people. One important trend is the move towards mobile or remote wardens as a means of avoiding large-scale capital costs, reported in eleven schemes. Stockport Housing Department (1980) estimated that sheltered housing new build costs about twelve times more per dwelling than a mobile alarm system, although the benefits of a mobile warden may also be less than those of an on-site warden.

Finance

Schemes reported three main sources of finance for housing innovations: SSD base budget (sixteen reports), the housing department base budget (fifteen reports) and joint finance (ten reports). Many housing departments believe sheltered housing to be a costly resource 'carried' by general needs housing. However, the use of joint finance as a means of financing very sheltered housing seems more widespread than suggested by Butler, Oldman and Grieve (1983) who argued that the incompatibility between the Department of the Environment and the Department of Health and Social Security subsidy systems would pose formidable administrative difficulties.

Organisational process

There seem to be two main reasons given for the development of very sheltered housing schemes, each indicating an incentive for SSD and housing departments to co-operate. Fifteen reports mentioned pressure on Part III (an incentive for SSDs to collaborate), while eighteen mentioned service failure, usually within mainstream sheltered housing (an incentive for housing departments to co-operate). The initiating personnel were similarly likely to be drawn either from the housing department (nine reports), the SSD (seven reports) or a joint group (eleven reports). Co-operation at planning level thus seems firmer than co-operation at operational level (Bytheway and James, 1978), reflecting a potentially symmetrical pattern of incentives for planning staff within the two agencies.

The strength of innovatory pressures should not be overstated, as the sector was significantly less likely than the rest of the sample to report successful replication (Table 7.1). Nine reports indicated that schemes were still proceeding on pilot money, and only five reported transition to post-pilot status. A majority (23) had been started within the last five years so were still at an early stage of historical development.

A substantial risk in many of these schemes is that they will become resource intensive 'showcase' programmes which are incapable of replication on an authority-wide basis. Only Warwickshire appears to be pursuing a coherent district-by-district approach to the implementation of a county-wide, very sheltered housing programmme.

A final theme concerns the pattern of joint working in the schemes. Not only is this crucial to agreed allocation policies but it could influence the present debate about the low transfer rates from sheltered housing to residential or nursing homes. Although these may reflect success in reducing the need for transfers, a more likely explanation is that there are insufficient joint links to ensure that the vacancies which do arise are offered to sheltered housing tenants (Heumann and Boldy, 1982). Fourteen schemes reported some form of joint working with the NHS, a similar proportion to the rest of the sample. Liaison with social workers and the home help service represented the strongest channels of external contact.

Another form of joint working consists of community development within the schemes. A criticism frequently made of sheltered housing concerns the lack of social interaction in the facilities. Page and Muir (1971) suggested that conventional sheltered housing provision did not succeed in socially engaging isolated tenants. An important theme within very sheltered housing has been the alteration of organisational arrangements so as to enhance social interaction. The evaluation of the Warwickshire programme (Warwickshire SSD, 1980) commented that relieving the burden of the warden seemed to be associated with an increase in the amount of social activity. Whereas in the mainstream sheltered schemes there was an average of 1.75 social activities per week, for the very sheltered schemes this figure had risen to six. Furthermore, more of the schemes in the very sheltered programme were organised by the tenants themselves as opposed to wardens or volunteers. Thus almost half (fifteen) the schemes in the housing sector reported such community development work, most frequently through the provision of improved day-care facilities. However, there was only one report of involvement of informal carers and none of neighbourly help, so in many ways the isolation of the schemes from informal help continues.

In conclusion, the argument that very sheltered housing could act as an extra point on the continuum of care is widely but not totally accepted. Some housing authorities continue to define the problem in housing terms, whereas others advocate a counter movement based on sheltering at home. Nevertheless there is now a rapid development of Category 2 schemes. A major problem consists of the lack of case management at tenant level as the evidence suggests a picture of incremental additions to particular services rather than the introduction of powerful case managers. The neglect of case management can be seen in the low priority given to assessment, care packaging and service arranging, and the provision of direct work. The role of the lay warden has continued to lag behind the extra demands placed upon it. This failure to develop explicit co-ordinating mechanisms is especially surprising given that the use of joint finance is much more extensive than previous work has suggested.

Case Studies

The commentary has already drawn attention to the variety of new services now being developed. This can be demonstrated more clearly by a closer look at three distinct schemes: 'extensive' sheltered housing, 'intensive' sheltered housing and community-based warden services.

Birmingham Housing Department: Vertical Warden Scheme

This 'extensive' form of sheltered housing illustrates how property that could be unpopular with other client groups can be adapted at low cost to produce new sheltered housing units.

In common with many housing-based schemes, attention was not given to developing enhanced referral mechanisms. Table 7.2 illustrates the desire to improve uptake by a programme of rapid expansion, only possible in the case of low-cost adaptation of existing property.

Little emphasis was placed on case management characteristics: these schemes are not designed for highly dependent tenants. Table 7.3 shows that as part of the conversion process warden cover was provided, together with a two-way speech alarm system connected to the warden's flat and a restrictive access entry communication system. No extra care inputs were made available.

The contribution of extensive sheltered housing in increasing service efficiency lies first of all in reducing the need for residential and hospital care and in providing extra units at low cost. As the scheme was housing department financed, it is not surprising that objectives such as the alleviation of underoccupation and of overoccupation take precedence over objectives traditionally associated with SSDs, such as the provision of short-term care, rehabilitation or support for informal carers (Table 7.4).

Housing department staff introduced the scheme in response to continuing high demand from elderly people (Table 7.5). The pilot scheme was evaluated as successful and replication is being considered in new types of accommodation such as low-rise flats and bungalows. As far as joint working is concerned, the only noticeable feature was the provision of communal facilities in order to eliminate the isolation often associated with multistorey living (Table 7.6).

153

Table 7.2
Birmingham Housing Department
Vertical Warden Scheme:
case finding

Dimension	Response
Targeting (eligibility criteria)	No/no mention
Targeting (client subgroups)	No/no mention
Uptake	Intention to raise uptake, e.g. introduction of free service, creation of more accessible resources
Outreach	No/no mention
Referral process	No/no mention
Preventive surveillance	No/no mention

Table 7.3
Birmingham Housing Department
Vertical Warden Scheme:
case management

Dimension	Response
Assessment (type)	No/no mention
Assessment (inputs)	No/no mention
Care packaging (type)	No/no mention
Care packaging (scope)	No/no mention
Arranging for additional services	No/no mention
Direct work	No/no mention
Monitoring (type)	No/no mention
Monitoring (scope)	No/no mention
Monitoring (by whom?)	No/no mention
Improved communications	Speech link to resident warden Entry communication
Key worker (role)	No/no mention
Key worker (who?)	No/no mention

154

Table 7.4
Birmingham Housing Department
Vertical Warden Scheme:
efficiency

Dimension	Response
Short-term commitment	No/no mention
Rehabilitation	No/no mention
Lower-cost mode	Shift from institutional care
Support for informal carers	No/no mention
More efficient production process	Low-cost adaptations
Source of finance	Housing department

Table 7.5
Birmingham Housing Department
Vertical Warden Scheme:
organisational process

Dimension	Response
Problem context	Demographic trends
Initiating personnel	Housing department staff
Pilot?	Post-pilot phase
Duration	Less than 5 years
Coverage	Several schemes

Conclusion 'Extensive' sheltered housing schemes show few of the case-finding and case management characteristics associated with many SSD-based schemes for the more dependent elderly. Emphasis is on the rapid expansion of low-cost provision rather than catering for the more frail elderly.

Wealden District Council: The Polegate Project

This is an example of 'intensive' sheltered housing, incorporating both social and health care inputs. However, concern is also shown for

155

Table 7.6
Birmingham Housing Department
Vertical Warden Scheme:
joint working

Dimension	Response
Joint working (SSD staff)	No/no details
Joint working (NHS staff)	No/no details
Volunteers/voluntary organisations	No/no details
Housing staff	No/no details
Community development	Improved day centre/club facilities
Evaluation (by implementors)	No/no details
Evaluation (by other internal officers)	Yes – unspecified
Evaluation (by external evaluators)	No/no details

voluntary activities and community development, the whole site being planned as a joint exercise throughout.

The scheme caters for the more dependent elderly on the margin of either admission to, or discharge from, hospital or residential care (Table 7.7). However, great emphasis is also placed on voluntary as well as statutory day care activities, identifying elderly isolated people

Table 7.7
Wealden District Council Polegate Project:
case finding

Dimension	Response
Targeting (eligibility criteria)	On margin of need for residential care/frail/at risk Post-discharge care
Targeting (client subgroups)	No/no mention
Uptake	No such intention/mention
Outreach	Socially isolated
Referral process	No/no mention
Preventive surveillance	No/no mention

in the community who could benefit from day centre attendance and organising the necessary transport.

A variety of services are available, although there are no reports of joint assessments or of explicit powers to arrange new combinations of service which might indicate more elaborate forms of care planning. The appointment of a community services officer, however, is meant to ensure that health, social service and housing inputs are linked together, thus undertaking a key worker and co-ordinating role (Table 7.8). Individual and group counselling facilities are available for tenants and relatives, in addition to a warden service with an enhanced care component in the job description.

No report was received of building to enhanced design standards. However, care assistants provided domestic and personal care, and skilled nursing care was available from a full-time district nursing sister attached to the project.

The project pursues greater efficiency in a number of ways. Within a linked Part III home, six short-term beds are set aside to form a short-term special intensive care unit (Table 7.10). It would take clients, say, who had fallen or who had bronchitis, thus avoiding the necessity for admission to hospital through rehabilitative work. Support for informal carers is available through support groups and

Table 7.8
Wealden District Council Polegate Project:
case management

Dimension	Response
Assessment (type)	No/no mention
Assessment (inputs)	No/no mention
Care packaging (type)	General commitment
Care packaging (scope)	SSD residential care
	NHS community services
	Sheltered housing
Arranging for additional services	No/no mention
Direct work	With client
Monitoring (type)	No/no mention
Monitoring (scope)	No/no mention
Monitoring (by whom?)	No/no mention
Improved communications	Enhanced warden cover
Key worker (role)	Co-ordination
Key worker (who?)	Co-ordinating post

Table 7.9
Wealden District Council Polegate Project:
care provision

Dimension	Response
Enhanced physical facilities	No/no mention
Domestic care	General commitment
Personal care	General commitment
Nursing care	Skilled nursing care
Specialist care (eligibility criteria)	On margin of need for institutional care
	Post-discharge care
Specialist care (client subgroups)	No/no mention

active use is made of volunteers in community development tasks. The scheme is financed in part by the housing department, with 100 per cent joint finance secured for the staff costs in the first instance, with subsequent reviews.

The scheme has been conceived and implemented by a joint working party including health, housing, social services and voluntary representatives. It is seen as a three-year experiment to test a possible pattern for future development, involving a wide range of personnel

Table 7.10
Wealden District Council Polegate Project:
efficiency

Dimension	Response
Short-term commitment	Relief care
Rehabilitation	Physical rehabilitation
Lower-cost mode	Shift from institutional care
	Support for informal carers
	Use of volunteers
Support for informal carers	Relatives' support group
More efficient production process	No/no mention
Source of finance	Joint finance
	Housing department

from various agencies as well as enhanced day care services (Table 7.11).

Conclusion Intensive sheltered housing schemes may well produce a greater number and variety of care inputs, yet the number of residents benefiting from such schemes is small and the planning process demanding.

Hammersmith and Fulham Housing Department: sheltering at home

With enhanced alarm systems, councils are increasingly able to offer many of the benefits of sheltered housing to elderly people remaining in their homes, enabling them to remain within a particular locality and avoiding the capital costs associated with conventional provision.

The main contribution made to case finding lies in the provision of a community alarm service to a group of elderly people, many of whom are at risk. Half the participants in the scheme had had accidents in their home within the last year. Each pensioner has a small matchbox-sized unit, with a button to be pressed in case of a fall, sending out a message to a call-in telephone number.

The scheme, unlike many housing-based innovations, displays a number of case management features. Table 7.13 indicates that allocation is dependent on an overall, domiciliary-based assessment of housing, health and social factors. Only about one-third of applications are successful. As well as providing mobile warden cover, the area warden is also expected to advise on any housing adaptations, repairs or improvements advisable. About 50 per cent of clients are public sector tenants, about 25 per cent owner occupiers and 25 per cent private tenants. There were no reports of out-of-hours working or of key workers explicitly responsible for planning packages of provision.

The project emphasises the contribution improved housing standards can make to enabling elderly people to stay in their homes and home areas. The warden provides surveillance, but extra SSD or health inputs are not allocated directly to the scheme.

The priority of the scheme lies in producing low-cost housing resources rather than social care: there is no reported use of volunteers, rehabilitation or support for families. Finance came from the housing department and through the Inner Areas Programme (Table 7.15).

Table 7.16 again indicates the marginal nature of many schemes funded by external finance. The pilot phase is also being carefully monitored. As far as relationships with other agents are concerned, the area warden is careful to maintain close relationships with local

Table 7.11
Wealden District Council Polegate Project:
organisational process

Dimension	Response
Problem context	Pressure on OPH beds
	Demographic trends
Initiating personnel	Joint working: JCPT/joint central NHS/SSD committee
Pilot?	Yes
Duration	Less than 5 years
Coverage	One scheme
Joint working (SSD staff)	Social workers
Joint working (NHS staff)	Nurses/nursing officers
	GPs
	OTs
Volunteers/voluntary organisations	General commitment
Housing department staff	Wardens
Community development	Improved day centre/club facilities
Evaluation (by implementors)	No/no details
Evaluation (by other internal officers)	Yes – unspecified
Evaluation (by external evaluators)	No/no details

Table 7.12
Hammersmith and Fulham housing
department sheltering at home:
case finding

Dimension	Response
Targeting (eligibility criteria)	No/no mention
Targeting (client subgroups)	No/no mention
Uptake	Community-based alarm systems
Outreach	No/no mention
Referral process	No/no mention
Preventive surveillance	No/no mention

Table 7.13
Hammersmith and Fulham housing department sheltering at home: case management

Dimension	Response
Assessment (type)	Focus on problems/strengths rather than eligibility for service Assessment at home
Assessment (inputs)	SSD staff NHS staff Housing department staff
Care packaging (type)	No/no mention
Care packaging (scope)	No/no mention
Arranging for additional services	Innovation in formal procedure for arranging other services by agencies other than the SSD
Direct work	No/no mention
Monitoring (type)	No/no mention
Monitoring (scope)	No/no mention
Monitoring (by whom?)	No/no mention
Improved communications	Central call-in system Community-based alarms
Key worker (role)	No/no mention
Key worker (who?)	No/no mention

Table 7.14
Hammersmith and Fulham housing department sheltering at home: care provision

Dimension	Response
Enhanced physical facilities	General commitment
Domestic care	No/no mention
Personal care	No/no mention
Nursing care	No/no mention
Specialist care (eligibility criteria)	No/no mention
Specialist care (client subgroups)	Falls

161

Table 7.15
Hammersmith and Fulham housing department sheltering at home: efficiency

Dimension	Response
Short-term commitment	No/no mention
Rehabilitation	No/no mention
Lower-cost mode	Shift from institutional care
Support for informal carers	No/no mention
More efficient production process	Low-cost adaptations
Source of finance	Inner Areas Project
	Housing department

Table 7.16
Hammersmith and Fulham housing department sheltering at home: organisational process

Dimension	Response
Problem context	Observed failure of present service: disregard of client preferences
	Budgetary pressures
Initiating personnel	Housing department staff
	Joint working: other central group/corporate key issue review
Pilot?	Yes
Duration	Less than 5 years
Coverage	One scheme
Joint working (SSD staff)	Social workers
Joint working (NHS staff)	No/no mention
Volunteers/voluntary organisations	No/no mention
Housing department staff	Wardens
	Housing action area staff
Community development	Improved day centre/club facilities
Evaluation (by implementors)	No/no details
Evaluation (by other internal officers)	Yes – unspecified
Evaluation (by external evaluators)	No/no details

162

social workers. Work with the NHS or voluntary organisations is not mentioned. The project has provided communal facilities similar to those in sheltered housing by using a new local community centre.

8 Innovation in the Voluntary Sector

Commentary

This chapter discusses the 28 voluntary sector schemes contained in Ferlie, Challis and Davies (1983), again taking more detailed written reports of these schemes from Ferlie (1982). Up to this point we have only considered public sector innovations, yet the role of the voluntary sector may also be important. One argument is that the voluntary sector pioneers new forms of service which are then legitimised and replicated within public sector mainstream programmes. For instance, Gladstone (1979) argues that the role of the voluntary sector should be further expanded due to its greater capacity for 'innovation' and 'flexibility', citing preventive and co-ordinative work as well as support for informal carers as examples of such pioneering potential. Other writers have questioned the validity of this general assumption: Schorr (1970) argues that the most significant developments in American social policy in the 1960s were government led, with marginal connections with voluntary services.

The character of the voluntary sector has clearly changed over time. Thus the Wolfenden Report (1978) concluded that since 1950 the number of voluntary organisations has rapidly expanded, with growth concentrated among organisations catering, often on a mutual aid basis, for specific client groups and among organisations concerned to influence policies as well as to provide services. The traditional philanthropic role of voluntary organisations, however, has declined

164

over time. Voluntary organisations may also have functions within an increasingly differentiated public sector as improvers and advocates as well as direct service providers. *The Rising Tide* (Health Advisory Service, 1983) thus referred to the role of Age Concern and MIND as pressure groups influencing the development of public psychogeriatric services. In its examination of this issue, the Wolfenden Report concluded by commenting that voluntary provision should be extended:

> Where the voluntary sector possesses advantages by way of specialist knowledge and skills and flexibility; and as an encouragement to voluntary organisations to make well judged entries into those fields where, without a wasteful use of capital resources, a leavening of choice and variety could be introduced (1978, p.188).

The style of a voluntary organisation is crucial and has a pervasive influence on the nature of innovatory schemes launched. Young (1976) outlines the different management styles open to non-profit agencies, one of which is termed 'innovative elitist'. Such agencies emphasise professional recognition as a key objective with a tendency to undertake a variety of 'showcase' programmes in response to governmental requests which ensure that such demonstration projects conform closely to public sector priorities.

The child care field contains a range of innovative/elitist agencies such as the New York child care agencies studied by Young and Finch (1977) which displayed a sense of mission rather than the conventional patterns of goal displacement found in large-scale organisations, with new goals replacing old as the number of children in residential care declined. In the care of elderly people such innovative/elitist organisations are less well established (replicating a public sector division of prestige) but Age Concern and MIND represent the best examples of professionalised agencies with specialist central support staff. In terms of agency characteristics, these organisations are large-scale, formalised (at least above front-line level) and professionalised. Dependence on soft-money public sector grants increases the power of the technostructure within the agency which has the technical bargaining skills required. This erosion of agency independence may serve to align voluntary sector and public sector priorities. As Kramer concludes in his review of American funding arrangements:

> Grantmanship, the know-how required to obtain time-limited funds for a special purpose — research, demonstration, facility construction, or a service program for a particular agency — has become a fiscal way of life for most public service organisations in the United States. As a result, governmental and voluntary agencies are becoming more like

each other because of their dependency on a grants economy with multiple funding sources in the 'banker' state and federal government, as well as in private foundations (1981, p.156).

Age Concern represents a good example of such a voluntary agency undertaking promotional and developmental work on a client group basis. Founded in 1940 as the National Old People's Welfare Committee (the change of name took place in 1971) Age Concern has now built up 1,300 groups and claims 115,000 volunteers. Local Age Concern groups now deliver a range of services (Dickson, 1980) including sheltered housing, health education, hospital aftercare, stroke clubs and day care for elderly mentally infirm people. Recent national initiatives include Age Concern's Action Against Crime campaign which provided small grants to pump prime Victim Support Schemes. Age Concern (1981) reports a collection of local initiatives in the provision of services for elderly mentally infirm people and their relatives and further urges local groups to press for the improvement of public facilities through, for example, the appointment of a psychogeriatrician in each health district.

There are two areas in which innovative voluntary sector provision complementing public sector provision might most fruitfully develop. The first is community-based care for elderly mentally infirm people. Dartington (1978) argues that psychiatric aftercare is an area in which voluntary organisations are well equipped to help those accorded low priority by the public sector and those on the margins of two very different formal systems, social care and health care. Norman (1982) notes the rapid growth of voluntary specialist day centres offering support for clients varying from those suffering from severe dementia to socially isolated elderly people, but also draws attention to the key role of the paid organiser or professional in establishing such initiatives and in training and supporting volunteers in developing specialist knowledge. A second complementary role of voluntary provision could be to offer relief to informal carers: Hatch (1980, p.101) argues that the participatory character of many voluntary organisations, particularly the mutual aid groups, gives the voluntary sector advantages in better access to the informal sector, although this may not be the case in bureaucratised and formalised voluntary agencies anxious to mimic the public sector.

A related area concerns the development of neighbourhood care. During the 1970s, there was renewed interest in the promotion of 'good neighbouring' resulting in the DHSS-sponsored launch of a Good Neighbour campaign in 1976. Abrams, Abrams, Humphrey and Snaith (1981) found that the neighbourhood schemes surveyed worked with elderly people more than any other client group: 82 per cent reported serving elderly people as opposed to only 11 per cent young families. The main contribution of the schemes was towards the light end of the spectrum, including such tasks as monitoring. The major problems faced by neighbourhood schemes were found to be based on shortage of helpers (43 per cent) and 'inappropriate helpers' (21 per cent). Middle-class volunteers could find it difficult to befriend working-class clients. In addition neighbourhood-based schemes may not accept public agency-based definitions of efficiency but rather value their autonomy and pursue localist goals. In contrast professionals may wish to reduce the autonomy of the neighbourhood group by controlling patterns of referral. So reports from neighbourhood schemes need to be analysed for contributions to target efficiency, for reports of difficulty of recruitment and for the extent of linkage with the public sector.

Vertical target efficiency

First, the targeting arrangements reported by voluntary sector schemes which affect vertical target efficiency are examined. Previous evidence suggests poor vertical targeting in the voluntary sector. Hadley, Webb and Farrell (1975) found that 37 per cent of their sample of those receiving a volunteer had a 'low need' for visiting, a figure confirmed by Shenfield and Allen (1972). This poor performance was seen as due to inadequate assessment and allocation procedures.

Only nine of the 28 voluntary sector schemes reported any arrangements for targeting by eligibility criteria, a significantly lower proportion than the rest of the sample (Table 8.1). On the other hand the sector was significantly more likely to target by client subgroup than the rest of the sample, with emphasis on elderly mentally infirm people (fourteen schemes) and relative support (nine schemes). This discrepancy could be because at least some of the criteria in the first dimension relate to essentially administrative definitions (the margin of admission to residential care or post-discharge support), whereas those in the second definition are based on subgroup-based need concepts which voluntary agencies may find easier to serve. This evidence points to a complementary division of labour between the public and voluntary sectors, with the latter concentrating efforts on two priority subgroups.

Horizontal target efficiency

The voluntary sector is often seen as placing high emphasis on uptake and outreach. Thus the Wolfenden Report (1978, p.28) argues that

167

Table 8.1
Signs of efficiency improvement:
voluntary sector compared with other sectors

Sign	Chi square	Direction
1. Targeting (eligibility criteria)	4.57**	negative
2. Targeting (client subgroups)	9.51***	positive
3. Uptake	0.37	positive
4. Outreach	25.64***	positive
5. Assessment (enhanced type)	2.15	negative
6. Assessment (multidisciplinary)	3.63*	negative
7. Care packaging	3.64*	positive
8. Service arranging	4.33**	negative
9. Direct work	1.98	positive
10. Monitoring/follow-up	1.95	negative
11. Key worker	4.60**	negative
12. Personal care	0.04	negative
13. Night sitting	(not computed)	
14. Out-of-hours working	5.68**	negative
15. Short-term working	20.32***	negative
16. Rehabilitation	0.48	negative
17. Shift from institutional care	13.48***	negative
18. Support for informal carers	4.18**	positive
19. More efficient production process	9.84***	positive
20. Joint finance	2.87*	negative
21. Replication	5.38**	negative
22. Joint working with NHS	0.04	positive

Notes
* p at .10
** p at .05
*** p at .01
Source: Ferlie et al. (1984).

the voluntary sector is the ideal medium for spontaneous and speedy action. However, the evidence suggests that the proportion of voluntary schemes reporting better uptake was almost exactly the same as the rest of the sample (Table 8.1). But the voluntary sector was much more likely than the rest of the sample to report outreach activity, particularly in the case of elderly mentally infirm people (fourteen reports) (Table 8.1). For example the Sheffield Northern General Project Home Care Relief Pilot (Ferlie, 1982) aims at supporting those at home who care for elderly patients discharged from a psychogeriatric ward. It began as a result of concern about the discharge of elderly severely mentally frail patients to the care of relatives who did not qualify for SSD domiciliary support. The aim of the project is to enable the families to cope with their difficult situation and also to prevent or delay further hospital admissions.

Other signs of horizontal target efficiency were accorded little prominence by the voluntary sector schemes. For instance only six schemes mentioned enhancements to the referral process to improve the flow of cases. Only five reported preventive surveillance functions, indicating that schemes organised by formal voluntary organisations such as Age Concern and MIND are likely to be facility rather than community centred. They may well display rather more similarities with public sector schemes than neighbourhood care schemes, which Abrams et al. (1981) argue are more likely to emphasise community-based preventive surveillance.

Case management

It might be thought that voluntary sector schemes would display low emphasis on case management tasks. Shenfield and Allen (1972) and Hadley, Webb and Farrell (1975) both drew attention to the lack of emphasis on assessment skills and the tendency to go for quantity rather than quality in service provision. Although the voluntary sector was somewhat less likely than the rest of the sample to report an enhanced type of assessment, the difference was not significant (Table 8.1). On the other hand schemes in the voluntary sector were significantly less likely to report provision for a multidisciplinary approach to assessment (Table 8.1), illustrating the danger of isolation in the delivery of care services. It was clearly difficult for voluntary schemes to undertake care packaging and indeed only two schemes in the sector reported such activity. Only one scheme reported enhanced service arranging in collaboration with a public agency. Thus the pluralism commended by Wolfenden (1978) as a hallmark of a service system containing a strong voluntary component may also result in intersectoral service fragmentation which makes the delivery of a co-ordinated package of care to clients more difficult to achieve.

One 'sign' in the case management sector is now discussed where the voluntary sector performed perhaps surprisingly well: direct work. Although the difference was not significant, voluntary sector schemes were slightly more likely than the rest of the sample to report direct work activity (Table 8.1). In some of these schemes, such as the Age Concern (Wandsworth) Counselling Groups (Ferlie, 1982), there was evidence that the voluntary sector was acting as a pioneer in responding to newly legitimised needs such as bereavement counselling. This scheme operated in partnership with the public sector, receiving DHSS funding. In other schemes volunteers were able to maintain intensive, long-term, one-to-one involvement which would not have been possible in the public sector due to staff constraints. Volunteer stroke schemes run by the Chest, Heart and Stroke Association represent a good example of such an approach (Eaton Griffith and Miller, 1980).

Other signs confirmed the lack of emphasis on case management within the voluntary sector, reflecting lack of interest in accountability mechanisms. Only four schemes in the sector reported any kind of monitoring system. None reported any arrangement for audit or review of services. None reported any key worker system, a sign which showed a strong negative association with voluntary sector status (Table 8.1). If the voluntary sector is to assume greater importance in the care of elderly people, then these weaknesses will become target areas for improvement.

Service content

The voluntary sector did not perform well on the signs of service content. It was no more likely than the rest of the sample to provide personal care (Table 8.1) and significantly less likely to report out-of-hours working (Table 8.1): rhetoric about sectoral 'flexibility' should be subjected to closer examination.

Cost-related criteria

Table 8.1 suggests that the voluntary sector does not focus on narrow bed-unblocking objectives. It was significantly less likely than the rest of the sample to report short-term working or a shift from institutional care. It seems instead to have a more diffuse, complementary role in providing care for subgroups accorded low priority by the public sector, such as support for relatives (Table 8.1). In the seventeen schemes in the voluntary sector which reported the provision of support for relatives in the voluntary sector, the tasks most frequently mentioned were individual volunteer support (eight schemes), relatives' support groups (seven schemes) and day care (five schemes). The clustering of localised day care schemes and relatives' support group schemes within the voluntary sector represents areas in which formal care provided by public bureaucracies may well face severe difficulties in interweaving with idiosyncratic and individually variable caring patterns.

Another efficiency advantage often claimed for the voluntary sector lies in its emphasis on rehabilitation. The potential is there, it is argued, for continuing one-to-one rehabilitative working. Yet it was found that the voluntary sector reported rehabilitative working in almost exactly the same proportion as the rest of the sample, with

170

effort concentrated on providing coping mechanisms for elderly mentally infirm people.

The voluntary sector is argued to provide better 'value for money' (Hatch and Mocroft, 1979), although intersectoral cost comparisons need to take adequate account of confounding factors such as client dependency and scale of operation. Interestingly, Knapp and Missiakoulis (1982) found voluntary day care units to be characterised by diseconomies of scale, although statutory units displayed economies of scale. The cost advantage to the voluntary sector may be then confined to smaller-scale facilities.

As far as a more efficient production process is concerned, the voluntary sector was significantly more likely to report activity than the rest of the sample (Table 8.1). Although there were no reports of the removal of diseconomies of scale (the small-scale production advantage argument), there were a number of reports of activity on the 'human capital' side, namely training of staff (five schemes) and management support (six schemes). These attempts to develop voluntary facilities which are skilled in terms both of manpower and management skills reflect a complementary model of provision where the voluntary sector is taking on skilled tasks neglected by the public sector. In these circumstances the voluntary sector can no longer afford to sacrifice quality to quantity.

It was instructive to note the source of finance for voluntary sector schemes. The Wolfenden Report (1978, p.168) argued that there was evidence of a substantial real rise in central government support for voluntary organisations which offset a relative decline in private giving. Such expansion was in turn most evident where government recognised that a voluntary organisation was an appropriate instrument for a particular policy — for example, the Home Office's support for NACRO. Such changes in the funding of voluntary organisations lend credence to the view that a complementary division of labour between the two sectors may be emerging.

Analysing the 28 voluntary sector schemes reported in Ferlie, Challis and Davies (1983) showed there were nineteen reports of voluntary organisation finance and five of trust finance. But there were also nineteen reports of public sector money going in, often SSD base budget money (six schemes) or joint finance (five schemes). Although such public sector finance might be expected to increase the level of voluntary sector alignment with public agency priorities, the voluntary sector reported significantly less use of joint finance than the rest of the sample (Table 8.1) which may help explain the lack of emphasis on bed-unblocking goals.

Voluntary sector schemes seem more likely to be launched in response to perceptions of (public sector) service failure (twelve schemes) than the more focused rationales of pressure on Part III (two reports only) or hospital beds (five reports) more commonly reported by public sector innovations. These schemes are overwhelmingly reported to have been initiated by voluntary sector personnel (24 reports) indicating that one should be careful not to overstate the degree of colonisation at least in terms of organisational process that takes place even in publicly-funded voluntary schemes. The availability of grants will certainly provide incentives to voluntary organisations to load their programmes in a particular direction, but public sector personnel are unlikely to undertake a detailed planning or monitoring role. Government evidence to the Wolfenden Report (1978, p.68) argued that in general the amount of detailed control which is exercised by departments over voluntary organisations to which grants are made is remarkably small.

Only a minority of voluntary sector schemes (six reports) indicated that they were at a pilot stage. However, there were other indicators of scheme marginality. For instance seventeen schemes reported a duration of less than five years, whereas only four reported a duration of more than five years. Voluntary sector schemes were significantly less likely to report replication than the rest of the sample (Table 8.1): the advantages of highly localist voluntary provision are paralleled by difficulties in effecting large-scale changes in voluntary sector provision.

The pattern of joint working reported by these schemes is also of interest. There was little joint working reported with housing departments (one scheme only). A minority of schemes reported joint working with the NHS (eleven schemes), where the occupational group most often mentioned consisted of nursing staff (five schemes), often in the context of work with elderly mentally infirm people. The proportion of schemes reporting joint work with the NHS was almost exactly the same as in the rest of the sample (Table 8.1). There were no reports of working with physiotherapists or occupational therapists, which indicates there is still further potential for development of the rehabilitative function of the voluntary sector. About half of the schemes (fifteen) reported joint working with SSD staff, most usually with social work staff. There was also a minority of schemes (nine) which reported community development work, reflecting a preference for autonomous action as opposed to colonisation.

Although only a minority of schemes (eight) reported any evaluative component, five involved universities or polytechnics out of a total of nine schemes contained in Ferlie, Challis and Davies (1983) which made provision for this type of evaluation. Lacking their own research capacity, innovative/elitist agencies have recourse to independent outside evaluators in order to examine the efficacy of important showcase programmes.

In conclusion, the voluntary schemes which made most contribution to the signs of efficiency were those launched by innovative/elitist agencies such as Age Concern and MIND. Although there were also a number of reports of neighbourhood care-based activity, schemes focused on the deployment of individual volunteers by social workers were notably absent. An emerging intersectoral division of labour was apparent, with the voluntary sector more likely to take on relative support and care for elderly mentally infirm people. At case level, coordinative mechanisms were weak. The tie-up with joint finance was also weaker than expected.

Case Studies

It has been argued that voluntary schemes may follow 'intensive' or 'extensive' models of service provision by focusing either on relationship work or on outreach activity. Two further dimensions relate to whether the scheme functions autonomously or in close collaboration with the statutory sector, and whether provision competes with or complements public social care. The following three case studies should indicate more clearly how these dimensions operate in practice.

Chest, Heart and Stroke Association: stroke rehabilitation

The scheme provides an example of the intensive use of volunteers in one-to-one work within schemes that are set up by the voluntary sector but which aim at enhancing public sector provision.

The schemes are aimed at improving the functioning and the quality of life of both discharged stroke patients and their families, the patient receiving weekly visits from each member of a small voluntary team and attending a weekly club (see Table 8.2). According to professional diagnosis, 93 per cent of clients had dysphasia, 45 per cent were considered to have severe speech problems and in 42 per cent comprehension was also affected (Table 8.3). The scheme is thus outreaching to heavily dependent people, the majority of whom are elderly.

As in many other voluntary schemes, few case management features are reported. However, for patients who have completed six months in the scheme, assessments are requested from the GP, speech therapist, family and volunteers. All agreed that 90–95 per cent of patients

Table 8.2
**Chest, Heart and Stroke Association
stroke rehabilitation:
case finding**

Dimension	Response
Targeting (eligibility criteria)	Post-discharge care
Targeting (client subgroups)	Stroke patients
	Support for relatives
Uptake	Intention to raise uptake, e g introduction of free service, creation of more accessible resources
Outreach	Stroke patients
Referral process	No/no mention
Preventive surveillance	No/no mention

**Table 8.3
Chest, Heart and Stroke Association
stroke rehabilitation:
case management**

Dimension	Response
Assessment (type)	No/no mention
Assessment (inputs)	OTs/physiotherapists
Care packaging (type)	No/no mention
Care packaging (scope)	No/no mention
Arranging for additional services	No/no mention
Direct work	With client
	With other informal carers
Monitoring (type)	Formal procedures on report-back on service adequacy
	Search for evidence beyond client self-reports
Monitoring (scope)	Voluntary inputs
Monitoring (by whom?)	GPs
	Volunteers
	Therapists
	Relatives
Audit/review?	No/no details
Key worker (role)	No/no mention
Key worker (who?)	No/no mention

showed general improvement and 70 per cent or more improved in speech. The volunteer undertakes a long-term relationship and rehabilitative work with stroke patients and also supports relatives. At the time of joining the scheme, 78 per cent of clients lived at home with their families, so family support is also an important task.

Although conventional care inputs (domestic care, personal care) are not supplied, rehabilitative work is undertaken in order to improve morale, social confidence and language recovery, and to support relatives (Table 8.4). As far as finance is concerned, the association's policy is to finance up to the first two years of a scheme, after which most health authorities have agreed to continue finance if the scheme has been successfully established. Payment is made to the association, which is responsible for maintaining standards.

This scheme is one in which the initiative came from the voluntary organisation itself: schemes have been set up in a wide variety of districts. Pilot schemes have evolved into long-running projects in various places.

The work is undertaken in collaboration with health services personnel such as a speech therapist but also promotes community development by setting up new voluntary groups and forms of day care (Table 8.5). An evaluation study has been published in the *British Medical Journal* (Eaton Griffith and Miller, 1980).

Age Concern (Gateshead): hospital aftercare

This scheme was designed in close collaboration with the NHS to provide a follow-up service unavailable in the public sector for discharged patients. Originally seen as an 'extensive' short-term service, it seems to be drifting towards a long-term basis as volunteers are reluctant to 'let go' of isolated elderly people.

The scheme is targeted on elderly people who could be discharged from hospital given greater domiciliary support (Table 8.6). The scheme worker negotiated direct access to referrals whereby daily telephone calls are made to hospital admissions clerks to establish any new admissions who might benefit from the scheme. If the patient is willing to accept help, he or she is visited and their needs are discussed with the ward sister and hospital social worker and a joint decision made about aftercare. The fieldworker keeps in touch with the ward to learn of the patient's condition and of any plans for discharge.

Apart from these joint decision-making procedures, the main case management features of the scheme are the co-ordinating role played by the voluntary organiser and the additional assessments carried out at home (Table 8.7). Other SSD or NHS services, however, are not

Table 8.4
Chest, Heart and Stroke Association
stroke rehabilitation:
efficiency

Dimension	Response
Short-term commitment	No/no mention
Rehabilitation	Stroke
Lower-cost mode	Support for informal carers
	Use of volunteers
Support for informal carers	Volunteers
More efficient production process	No/no mention
Source of finance	NHS base budget
	Voluntary organisation

Table 8.5
Chest, Heart and Stroke Association
stroke rehabilitation:
organisational process

Dimension	Response
Problem context	Observed failure of present service: inadequate case finding/uptake
Initiating personnel	Voluntary organisers
Pilot?	Post-pilot phase
Duration	More than 5 years
Coverage	Authority-wide/large-scale replication
Joint working (SSD staff)	No/no details
Joint working (NHS staff)	General commitment
Joint working (volunteers/ voluntary organisations)	Individual volunteers
Housing department staff	No/no details
Community development	Enhanced day care facilities
	Creation of new voluntary resources
Evaluation (by implementors)	No/no details
Evaluation (by other internal officers)	Yes – unspecified
Evaluation (by external evaluators)	No/no details

176

Table 8.6
Age Concern (Gateshead) hospital aftercare:
case finding

Dimension	Response
Targeting (eligibility criteria)	Post-discharge care
Targeting (client subgroups)	No/no mention
Uptake	No such intention/mention
Outreach	No/no mention
Referral process	Extension of post-admission assessment
	More direct access
Preventive surveillance	No/no mention

Table 8.7
Age Concern (Gateshead) hospital aftercare:
case management

Dimension	Response
Assessment (type)	No/no mention
Assessment (inputs)	Social workers
	Nursing staff
	Voluntary organisers
Care packaging (type)	No/no mention
Care packaging (scope)	No/no mention
Arranging for additional services	No/no mention
Direct work	With client
Monitoring (type)	No/no mention
Monitoring (scope)	No/no mention
Monitoring (by whom?)	No/no mention
Audit/review?	No/no details
Key worker (role)	Co-ordination
Key worker (who?)	Volunteers/voluntary organisers

available to be care packaged, nor is it clear how monitoring and audit functions are undertaken.

Volunteers are deployed in order to meet a broad range of needs, including medication and ensuring an adequate diet. Many clients reported social needs due to loneliness and isolation, and this has emerged as an important aspect of the project (Table 8.8).

Table 8.8
Age Concern (Gateshead) hospital aftercare:
care provision

Dimension	Response
Enhanced physical facilities	No/no mention
Domestic care	General commitment
Personal care	General commitment
Nursing care	No/no mention
Specialist care (eligibility criteria)	Post-discharge care
Specialist care (client subgroups)	Socially isolated

As Table 8.9 indicates, the scheme originally intended to offer help for a period of four to six weeks, although some of the clients have been given a service for much longer than the scheduled span. Rehabilitative work has included not only the restoration of social skills and independence but also the provision of support against isolation and loneliness. This support could also be used to relieve the pressure on families, as many elderly people in the scheme appeared to have had unrealistic expectations of the extent of family

Table 8.9
Age Concern (Gateshead) hospital aftercare:
efficiency

Dimension	Response
Short-term commitment	Post-discharge (hospital)
Rehabilitation	Social skills/independence
	Emotional support for anxiety/depression
Lower-cost mode	Shift from institutional care
	Support for informal carers
	Use of volunteers
Support for informal carers	Domiciliary care
	Volunteers
More efficient production process	No/no mention
Source of finance	Urban Aid
	Manpower Services Commission

178

care. There were no reports of the construction of adapted or low-cost provision often associated with the voluntary sector, in part because the scheme was not neighbourhood care-based but responding to specific NHS-defined needs. The scheme was delayed due to funding difficulties but finally proceeded under MSC and Urban Aid finance which supported the full-time fieldworker.

The initiative in setting up the project came from the appointment by Age Concern in 1977 of a development officer with a brief to investigate hospital aftercare services. Volunteer recruitment began in 1977 — there was no pilot stage — and the project started in 1978, taking referrals from a number of hospitals (Table 8.10), a broader field of coverage than found in many of the reported NHS schemes, which are restricted to a single hospital. The scheme involves consultations and joint assessments with both social services and NHS staff, and depends for its referrals on the hospital admissions records. The scheme also involves the recruitment of new volunteers as well as the efforts of an existing voluntary organisation. However, as this group

Table 8.10
Age Concern (Gateshead) hospital aftercare:
organisational process

Dimension	Response
Problem context	Pressure on hospital beds
	Demographic trends
	Pressure on NHS community services
Initiating personnel	Voluntary organisers
Pilot?	No/no mention
Duration	More than 5 years
Coverage	Authority-wide/large-scale replication
Joint working (SSD staff)	Social workers
Joint working (NHS staff)	Nurses/nursing officers
	GPs
Joint working (volunteers/voluntary organisations)	Individual volunteers
	Local branch of Age Concern
Housing department staff	No/no details
Community development	No/no details
Evaluation (by implementors)	No/no details
Evaluation (by other internal officers)	No/no details
Evaluation (by external evaluators)	University departments/units

was neither neighbourhood-based nor developed autonomy, it cannot be said that community development tasks were undertaken. Finally, a limited monitoring exercise was designed for the scheme in collaboration with the University of Newcastle.

Conclusion This scheme was designed to provide an extensive follow-up service in close collaboration with the NHS, with the aid of public finance. There appears to have been a drift to longer-term relationship work, changing the emphasis of the service offered.

Age Concern/MIND: Ormiston Road elderly mentally infirm day centre

This day centre for elderly mentally infirm people demonstrates the complementary role the voluntary sector can play in providing services for client groups traditionally given low priority by the public sector, with poor local public sector provision for both psychogeriatric services and specialist day care.

The scheme is closely targeted not only on clients themselves but also on offering relief and support to caring relatives. To this end the scheme not only provides extra local facilities but also outreaches to neglected elderly people or stressed relatives by providing care for the elderly person and close contact for relatives. No work, however, is done outside the day centre. One interesting feature is the relatively open referral policy in that referrals are accepted directly from relatives as well as professionals (Table 8.11).

The scheme provides for an initial domiciliary visit by either the MIND or Age Concern worker to assess the suitability of the person for the centre and vice versa (Table 8.12). Direct work is undertaken with clients on a one-to-one basis in an attempt to provide stimulation, and a relatives' support group has been formed, which meets two days a week to discuss access to other services, anxiety about coping with a confused person and the process of coming to terms with their relative becoming confused. There are, however, no reports of public services being available to care package along with these voluntary inputs. The workers complete daily assessments in order to provide monitoring, although more systematic audit or review mechanisms are not mentioned.

Apart from these general support functions, the only care service supplied is lunch, provided by the WRVS. As far as the relatives' support group is concerned, it is seen as important that workers and volunteers have lunch with the group.

The scheme contributes to service efficiency in a number of ways: by attempting at least to prevent deterioration in elderly confused

Table 8.11
Age Concern/MIND Ormiston Road
elderly mentally infirm day centre:
case finding

Dimension	Response
Targeting (eligibility criteria)	No/no mention
Targeting (client subgroups)	Elderly mentally infirm Support for relatives
Uptake	Intention to raise uptake, e.g. introduction of free service, creation of more accessible resources
Outreach	EMI/ESMI
Referral process	More direct access
Preventive surveillance	No/no mention

Table 8.12
Age Concern/MIND Ormiston Road
elderly mentally infirm day centre:
case management

Dimension	Response
Assessment (type)	Assessment at home
Assessment (inputs)	Voluntary organisers
Care packaging (type)	No/no mention
Care packaging (scope)	No/no mention
Arranging for additional services	No/no mention
Direct work	With client With other informal carers
Monitoring (type)	Set time intervals Search for evidence beyond client self-reports
Monitoring (scope)	Voluntary inputs
Monitoring (by whom?)	Volunteers Voluntary organisers
Audit/review?	No/no details
Key worker (role)	No/no mention
Key worker (who?)	No/no mention

**Table 8.13
Age Concern/MIND Ormiston Road
elderly mentally infirm day centre:
care provision**

Dimension	Response
Enhanced physical facilities	No/no mention
Domestic care	Preparation of meals
Personal care	No/no mention
Nursing care	No/no mention
Specialist care (eligibility criteria)	No/no mention
Specialist care (client subgroups)	Elderly mentally infirm
	Support for relatives

people; by using volunteers to support relatives and by providing improvised places at low cost in the local MIND centre, under voluntary finance (Table 8.14). There is, however, no report of short-term relief or rotating provision which might further increase the flexibility of the service.

**Table 8.14
Age Concern/MIND Ormiston Road
elderly mentally infirm day centre:
efficiency**

Dimension	Response
Short-term commitment	No/no mention
Rehabilitation	EMI coping strategies
Lower-cost mode	Support for informal carers
	Use of volunteers
Support for informal carers	Day care
	Volunteers
	Relatives' support group/counselling
More efficient production process	Low-cost adaptations
Source of finance	Voluntary organisation

Although the scheme was intended to fill 'gaps' in public provision, it emerged from the initiative of the two voluntary organisations concerned and is run in a managerially autonomous fashion (Table 8.15). It is of course limited in its coverage to one small area, as are many voluntary initiatives. However, further development may take place through the recently convened working party on the elderly mentally infirm on which the NHS and SSD are both represented. The scheme also represents an interesting development inside the voluntary sector in that new voluntary resources have been constructed jointly by two different voluntary organisations. The emphasis placed also on involving relatives in care can be seen as a form of community development. It would have been interesting to see the results of systematic evaluation as well as the limited monitoring exercise reported.

Table 8.15
Age Concern/Mind Ormiston Road
elderly mentally infirm day centre:
organisational process

Dimension	Response
Problem context	Observed failure of present service: inadequate case finding/uptake
Initiating personnel	Voluntary organisers
Pilot?	No/no mention
Duration	No details
Coverage	One district only
Joint working (SSD staff)	Social workers
Joint working (NHS staff)	General commitment
Individual volunteers/voluntary organisers	Individual volunteers recruited Local branches of voluntary organisations: Age Concern and MIND
Housing department staff	No/no details
Community development	Involvement of local volunteers/relatives in care
Evaluation (by implementors)	Yes
Evaluation (by other internal officers?)	No/no details
Evaluation (by external evaluators?)	No/no details

9 Conclusion

'Innovation', Change and Stagnation

Faced with a bewildering array of schemes all of which are defining change agendas slightly differently, it may well be thought that 'innovation' is a term without a coherent focus. Yet the achievement of a faster rate of qualitative change in service provision for the elderly is a major issue facing many human services organisations. Let us consider some of the themes which have emerged in the course of the study.

Drawing a map

The construction of a typology of innovation enables us to produce a map of this at first disorientating territory. The initial typology of efficiency improvement was found to be broader than the bulk of the schemes reported. Indeed a characteristic feature of the innovations reported was the narrow spectrum of activity: there was little joint working reported with the private and voluntary sectors (except for the publicly-sponsored large-scale pressure groups) and there were few reports of public sector interweaving with informal carers. Innovations designed to boost uptake or outreach or achieve greater technical efficiency (analogous to the cost improvement programme within the NHS) were conspicuous by their absence. The process of change was defined as internal to public agencies, centring on the achievement of narrow modal shift objectives. The broader implications of this will

184

be discussed in the second part of the chapter. There was a concentration on moves to personal care and case management roles in the personal social services, community-based working in the NHS and very sheltered housing in the housing sector. Voluntary agencies provided complementary services for groups accorded low priority by public sector agencies, such as the elderly mentally infirm and carers. Some schemes clearly make these shifts better than others: the distinction between typical and ideal schemes in each sector was explored in Ferlie, Challis and Davies (1984).

A theory of organisational change

Any analysis of organisation needs to go beyond cross-sectional studies to include a theory of change through time (Pettigrew, 1985). For all organisations, failure to adapt to changing conditions will lead to a decline in the organisation's performance which may or may not be remedied through corrective action, depending on the perceptions and leadership style of decision makers and the level of organisational resistance encountered. The inability to analyse processes of organisational change has been a major criticism of the organisational dimensions approach — in other ways so useful — associated with the Aston School. Such changes in environmental conditions are even more difficult to identify in human services organisations than in private sector firms because of the lack of such signals as falling profits or erosion of market share and the possibility of resorting to demand dampening devices such as waiting lists. But clearly the continuing rise in the numbers of very elderly and the fall-off in the growth rates enjoyed in the early 1970s represent major pressures for the adoption of input mix-centred innovation. The pressure for higher turnover within the NHS also has repercussions for SSDs and other community-based agencies. Changing professional ideologies (including increased professional interest in working with the elderly) and increased aversion to institutionally-based modes of care must also be considered as sources of change. The management of change assumes greater importance under conditions of greater instability (Burns and Stalker, 1961). Although the direction of change has been predictable, with the main lines of development apparent by the 1950s, the achievement of the new roles and models of service which make a community care policy possible are only now being worked through in a detailed way. Change at policy and increasingly at service level for mental health client groups has been far more rapid. The problem of engineering change is thus very real to human services organisations catering for elderly clients.

Since SSDs are isolated from direct consumer tests and provide a small areal monopoly able to enforce or withhold consumption, they lack many of the mechanisms which could stimulate performance review. Additionally their structure displays features of a mechanistic organisation seen as negatively associated with innovation. Thus Boaden (1971) argues that local government is marked by departmentalism, precise and risk-averse administration, strong line-management hierarchies and poor lines of communication. In no part of local government could these criticisms have been more valid than in the old welfare departments which placed much less emphasis on professional and developmental questions than children's departments. These complaints were reinforced when the failure to implement radical community care policies became apparent in the 1970s. Booth (1979) identified a number of conservative forces which made a policy of enhanced community care difficult: entrenched producer groups, an incremental budgetary procedure, the doctrine of *ultra vires*, the political preference for the construction of visible monuments such as new residential care facilities, the strength of the ratepayer lobby and a reluctance to take risks. In part this reflected a culture attuned to the equitable handling of cases and the lowering of the possibility of agency embarrassment, resulting in the displacement of more managerial conceptions of goal-directed behaviour.

Nevertheless departments develop reputations as 'sleepers' or 'thrusters' (Davies, Barton, McMillan and Williamson, 1971; Davies, Barton and McMillan, 1972; Lewis, 1976). An issue not considered in this book but analysed elsewhere is the identification of those factors associated with a higher SSD propensity to launch efficiency-improving innovation. Source of finance is one such characteristic. Ferlie, Challis and Davies (1985) found the use of joint finance to be associated with the achievement of a greater number of 'signs and symptoms' of efficiency improvement such as multidisciplinary assessment, enhanced post-discharge referral process or the provision of rehabilitation or new coping skills for the elderly mentally infirm. Base budget resource levels also appeared to exert an impact. Davies and Ferlie (1984) found that the degree of efficiency improvement reported in a data-base heavily weighted towards domiciliary care innovations was not related to changes in the overall measure of *per capita* expenditure on the elderly, but was positively related to increases in *per capita* home help expenditure. Although innovation was often based on input substitution objectives, and took place within a constrained macro financial climate, there was a requirement for a more favourable micro climate within the developing domiciliary care sector. Demographic pressure — the growth in the pensioner population — was also significantly related to the launching of externally financed innovation.

Previous work (Burns and Stalker, 1961) has argued that the degree of innovation achieved is likely to be greater in organisations with an 'organic' rather than a mechanistic role structure, with role fluidity, high levels of lateral communication, and reliance on task-working groups. Davies and Ferlie (1984) found evidence to suggest that such organisational features as a high measure of integration and a service review increased the likelihood of efficiency-improving innovation. A higher number of interdepartmental working groups was positively associated with internally-financed innovation, but a higher number of intradepartmental working groups was negatively associated with externally-financed innovation. Clearly the propensity to innovate is shaped by a complex mixture of financial, demographic and formal organisational characteristics, along with informal organisational and cultural factors which we were not able to explore in an extensive study.

Change processes

'Change' can of course take place in a number of ways. Organisational theories which make assumptions about goal-directed behaviour imply first, an element of purposiveness in the change process, and second that the process of change is managed within organisations, rather than taking place through market or quasi-market mechanisms. Both assumptions may be mistaken at least in the long term as professionally determined 'bottom-up' changes emerge over which the planning process has very little control. Firm style is a good example of such a bottom-up aspect of the process of change. Second, change can be directed by market signals as well as internal organisational processes. The far-reaching growth of publicly-financed private residential care which has made modal shift objectives more difficult to achieve was market rather than planning-based. This distinction between bureaucracies and markets as alternative modes of resource allocation leads to more general points about the analysis of alternative change processes.

Alternative policy models

The detailed information collected on over 200 schemes also contributes to more general policy arguments. Davies (1986) describes three models of a long-term care system for the elderly:

A The traditional British system of a few universalist, public, near monopolies with responsibility for financing, planning and provision of key forms of formal care.

B A mixed economy of welfare regulated to achieve minimal social objectives, containing a variety of public and non-public providers of care services. The public providers would not necessarily cover the greater part of the market. The formal care services could be provided and financed in a number of different ways including contracting out to the private sector, subject to regulation to prevent fraud, abuse and unwarranted escalation of costs. Much would also be financed privately with or without public subsidy and provided by non-public organisations. The financing mechanisms and provision would be subject to a lower degree of regulation than services, but regulated to avoid gross fraud or exploitation.

C A mixed economy of welfare led by public agencies with responsibility for developing and implementing a trade and industry policy for long-term care. This model differs from the second in the large and explicit role of lead public agencies. Such agencies would need to go beyond regulation to proactive identification of needs, and develop techniques to achieve change not only in the host lead agency but in other agencies. Davies (1986) argues that the adoption of the third rather than the second model rests on the identification of market failure, the demonstration of the insufficiency of retroactive regulation as a means of regulation, and the ability of traditionally risk-averse public agencies to take on the more entrepreneurial characteristics of the lead agency.

Each of the three policy models defines the main thrust of service innovation differently. Let us consider each in turn.

A. Public monopoly-dominated provision

The central problem in Model A is boundary management between the public near monopolies, and the substitution of less expensive SSD and housing forms of care for more expensive hospital forms of care. The cruder balance of care models emphasise the quantitative insufficiency of community care services. More sophisticated versions of the argument identify 'blockages' in the system which prevent optimal placement and overuse of high cost forms of provision. The creation of a large sheltered housing stock (and increasingly very sheltered housing) and new personal care and residential care roles reflects an emphasis within this model on the enhancement of service content. But as the public sector service system undergoes differentiation, so the search for integrative case management mechanisms even within the public sector becomes more acute. The management of post-hospital discharge arrangements has always been problematic, but the problem is sharpened by high turnover models of geriatric care and community-oriented psychogeriatric services. The growth of multidisciplinary 'teams' incorporating social and health care expertise is of increasing importance in these sectors, but such developments require the creation of team ideologies which legitimate shifts to role blurring and a more collegial style of working.

Most of the schemes reported in this study fall firmly within this Model A, yet most were targeted on incremental service content gains. There were few systematic attempts to improve the performance of case management tasks. There were some moves to multidisciplinary teams led by consultants, but apart from the community care projects (Davies and Challis, 1986), SSD-based case management schemes were conspicuously absent.

B. The American alternative

Model B poses a different set of issues not addressed by Model A, revolving around quality assurance. Such a perspective is of increasing interest in the British context given the recent expansion of the private sector: Laing (1985) estimates that private and voluntary homes will provide about 40 per cent of rest and nursing homes by 1990. Nevertheless there are continuing concerns about inequity, quality control and cost escalation in private sector systems which are residential care-led. Quality assurance is even more a concern in private sector-led systems than in public sector-led systems because of the regulators' lack of internal organisational control mechanisms. In particular there is a fear that the lack of screening for private sector entry will result in the admission of the less dependent and thus reverse modal shift, although Bebbington and Tong's (1986) evidence does not bear this out.

Private sector-based forms of provision are of growing but still limited importance in the United Kingdom. Private health insurance covered 1.6 million people in 1966 but 4.2 million in 1982, although this was often linked to company rather than individual purchase (Central Statistical Office, 1984) and covered acute rather than chronic illness. Private sector long-term care is thus funded through the social security programme rather than through insurance companies. However, financing responsibility has been divorced from regulatory responsibility and cost control has proceeded through crude budgetary caps and has been insensitive to local variations in the quality of care. Although the regulatory brief of SSDs has been expanded through recent legislation, even the best local authorities are only now feeling their way towards a regulatory framework. The screening of entry is one area where more rapid progress is now needed.

Another shift is the increasing transformation of at least some elderly people from clients allocated services by public sector decision makers acting 'on their behalf' into consumers spending their own resources. The personal disposable income of pensioners expressed as a proportion of that of non-pensioners has risen from 41 per cent in 1951 to 69 per cent in 1985 (Kay, 1985). This increase reflects both the growth of occupational pension schemes and improved state benefits. Over the next fifty years the incomes of the elderly, expressed as a percentage of the earnings of those at work, is projected to double (assuming no change in state earnings-related pensions schemes — SERPS) (Kay, 1985), mainly caused by the growth to maturity of occupational pensions schemes and SERPS.

Within Model B, consumers and private organisations retain considerable autonomy. If the public sector wishes to secure change, it could well be through the use of market signals rather than purposive organisational activity. In its most residual form, the public sector is left holding the ring in an attempt to prevent abuse. The American experience (Davies, 1986) suggests the following to be the crucial issues in this model of development: (i) the formulation of standards which are directly related to the quality of care; (ii) the design of a system able to assess compliance on a continuing basis; (iii) the implementation of effective enforcement mechanisms; and (iv) a reimbursement system which provides incentives for producers to increase the equity and efficiency of the long-term care system. In many ways the American system of financing tended to channel demand towards nursing homes and away from home and day care services, since Medicaid provided a straightforward supply of finance for nursing home care for the poor, while there was no corresponding source of finance for community-based alternatives.

C. Public lead agencies

Although there has been some erosion of the role of the public sector, a truly radical shift from public expenditure on social needs remains highly unlikely in the British context (Webb, 1985). The question which then arises is how this more pluralist system is to be co-ordinated. Model C presents a scenario in which public agencies take on a lead role. In this model although private and voluntary agencies have expanded the public sector has not withered away, providing less but retaining a dominant funding role. Although quality assurance in the publicly-financed private sector remains a key issue, as in Model B, such lead agencies have to address a number of other questions.

The development of case management roles not only within the public sector (as in Model A) but with the private, voluntary and informal

190

sectors The patch model of fieldwork organisation (Hadley and McGrath, 1984) takes a neighbourhood-based conception, focusing above all on locally-based kinship networks. Davies and Challis (1986) on the other hand describe a specialist team of social workers with delegated budgetary responsibility able to 'buy in' a wider range of resources operating in a retirement area with weak local kinship networks. The development of better case management (Davies, 1986) requires consideration of a number of themes: the implications of the form of field organisation adopted for tasks, skills and training; the definition of authority and responsibility; the use of devices such as delegated budgets or pooled funds; the creation of exchange relationships with personnel from other agencies; and collaboration of professionals with different backgrounds.

The use of public finances to secure social objectives in the subsidised voluntary sector In Model C, the public sector will fund a variety of service-providing voluntary agencies. Young's analysis (1976) of the regulation of non-profit organisations in the American context suggests that government can exert only limited pressure through the operation of economic incentives and political and administrative encouragement rather than coercion. The identification of sectors where the voluntary sector can best complement or substitute for public sector provision, the assessment of the relative quality of voluntary organisations bidding for public funds and the devising of funding mechanisms which are flexible enough to act as a monitoring tool yet long-term enough to ensure that voluntary organisations can devise stable plans are topics of particular interest.

A corporatist approach to the private sector Whereas the public sector retained a reactive role in its relationship with the private sector in Model B, it could also take on a more developmental brief by providing training and support for prospective proprietors, encouraging the formation of a proprietors' association with which it could negotiate and encouraging linkage through, for example, contracting out day care facilities.

British Social Care Maintenance Organisations (BRITSMOs) The BRITSMO entities (on the analogy of the US Social/Health Maintenance Organizations) would be publicly accountable, and subject to regulation by an entrepreneurial public agency responsible for leading the development of the local system (Davies, 1986). A core public agency would contract for services with other providers, under a contract obliging the provision of core services. The key case management role could be undertaken by the core public agency which could perform the case-finding functions not apparent in Model B.

Public entrepreneurs The core public agency within the BRITSMO would require an entrepreneurial management style both at operational and strategic levels. At street level the public agencies would require delegated powers and possibly decentralised budgets in order to adjust to small area variation in the balance of need and supply, to interweave effectively with other formal and informal providers, and to create a wider range of local resources. At strategic level, the development of a learning curve and the capacity to manage faster rates of change requires a shift from services (some of which may contain built-in obsolescence) to time-limited programmes which are subject to evaluation.

Conclusions

Each of the three models of development has different implications for strategies of service development. The third model in particular has yet to be explored fully. Each model has its own different logic of service development, distinguishing characteristic areas of activity in which innovation should be concentrated. This is not to imply a simplistic goal-directed conception of innovation: as well as sponsoring change directly, the centre may also seek to support bottom-up change which 'fits' with its chosen strategy. The important point is that the process of change should be strategically significant if the game of innovation is to be worth the candle.

References

Abrams, P. (1977), 'Community care: some research problems and opportunities', *Policy and Politics*, 6:2, 125–52.

Abrams, P., Abrams, S., Humphrey, R. and Snaith, R. (1981), *Action for Care: A Review of Good Neighbour Schemes in England*, The Volunteer Centre, Berkhamsted.

Age Concern (1972), *Role of the Warden in Grouped Housing*, Age Concern, London.

Age Concern (1980), *Hospital After Care Schemes*, Age Concern, London.

Age Concern (1981), *Mental Infirmity in Old Age*, Briefing 14(iv), Age Concern, London.

Aiken, M. and Hage, J. (1971), 'The organic organisation and innovation', *Sociology*, 5, 63–82.

Allen, I. (1982), *Short-stay Residential Care for the Elderly*, Policy Studies Institute, London.

Amos, G. (1973), *Care is Rare*, Age Concern, London.

Arie, T. (1975), 'Day care in geriatric psychiatry', *Gerontologica Clinica*, 17, 31–9.

Arie, T. and Isaacs, A.D. (1978), 'The development of psychiatric services for the elderly in Britain', in Isaacs, A.D. and Post, F. (eds), *Studies in Geriatric Psychiatry*, John Wiley, Chichester.

Arie, T. and Jolley, D. (1982), 'Making services work: Organisation and style of psychogeriatric services', in Levy, R. and Post, F. (eds), *The Psychiatry of Late Life*, Blackwell, Oxford.

Audit Commission (1985), *Managing Social Services for the Elderly More Effectively*, HMSO, London.

Audit Commission (1987), *Making a Reality of Community Care*, HMSO, London.

Audit Inspectorate (1983), *Social Services: Provision of Care for the Elderly*, HMSO, London.

Babbage, T. (1981), 'Sheltering the elderly in the community: Hammersmith's initiatives', *Housing Review*, May/June, 93.

Baker, F. (1983), 'Quality assurance and program evaluation', *Evaluation and the Health Professions*, 6:2, 149–60.

Barber, J.H. and Wallis, J.B. (1982), 'The effects of geriatric screening and assessment on general practice workload', *Health Bulletin*, 40:3, 125–32.

Barclay, P. (1982), *Social Workers: Their Role and Tasks*, Bedford Square Press, London.

Barrett, S. and Fudge, C. (1981), *Policy and Action*, Methuen, London.

Bayley, M. (1973), *Mental Handicap and Community Care*, Routledge and Kegan Paul, London.

Bayley, M. and Parker, P. (1980), 'Dinnington: An experiment in health and welfare cooperation', in Hadley, R. and McGrath, M. (eds), *Going Local*, Bedford Square Press, London.

Bebbington, A.C. (1979), 'Changes in the provision of social services to the elderly in the community over fourteen years', *Social Policy and Administration*, 13, 111–23.

Bebbington, A.C. and Davies, B.P (1983), 'Equity and efficiency in the allocation of the personal social services', *Journal of Social Policy*, 12:3, 309–31.

Bebbington, A.C., Davies, B.P., Charnley, H., Hughes, M., Ferlie, E. and Twigg, J. (1989), *Resources, Needs and Outcomes in Community-Based Care; A Comparative Study of Services for the Elderly in Ten Local Authorities*, Gower, Aldershot, forthcoming.

Bebbington, A.C. and Tong, M.S. (1986), 'Trends and changes in old people's homes: Provision over twenty years', in Judge, K. and Sinclair, I. (eds), *Residential Care for Elderly People*, HMSO, London.

Bedfordshire SSD (1978), 'Meals services in Bedfordshire', *Clearing House for Local Authority Social Services Research*, 2, 15–58.

Bergmann, K. (1978), 'Neurosis and personality disorder in old age', in Isaacs, A. and Post, F. (eds), *Studies in Geriatric Psychiatry*, Wiley, Chichester.

Bergmann, K. (1982), 'A community psychiatric approach to the care of the elderly: Are there opportunities for prevention?', in Magnussen, G. (ed.), *The Epidemiology and Prevention of Mental Illness in Old Age*, EGV, Hellerup, Denmark.

Bergmann, K., Foster, E.M., Justice, A.W. and Matthews, V. (1978), 'Management of the demented elderly patient in the community', *British Journal of Psychiatry*, 132, 441–9.

Boaden, N.T. (1971), 'Innovation and change in English local government', *Political Studies*, xix, 416–29.

Booth, T. (1979), 'Forward planning of local authority social services', in Booth, T. (ed.), *Planning for Welfare*, Blackwell, Oxford.

Booth, T., Barritt, A., Berry, S., Martin, D., Melotte, C. and Phillips, D. (1982), 'Dependency: Challenging the myths', *Community Care*, 21 October, 17–19.

Boucher, C.A. (1957), 'A survey of services available to the chronic sick and elderly in 1954–5', *Reports on Public Health and Medical Subjects*, 98, HMSO, London.

Brocklehurst, J.C. (1979), 'The development and present status of day hospitals', *Age and Ageing*, 8, Supplement, 79.

Brocklehurst, J.C. and Tucker, J.S. (1980), *Progress in Geriatric Day Care*, King Edward's Fund, London.

Brody, E.M. (1978), 'Community housing for the elderly: The program, the people, the decision-making process and the research', *The Gerontologist*, 18:2, 121–8.

Brotherton, J. (1975), *The Need for Meals-on-Wheels and Luncheon Clubs in the Dover District of Kent: Final Report*, Kent County Secretary's Department, Research and Intelligence Unit, Maidstone

Burley, L.E., Currie, C.T, Smith, R.G. and Williamson, J. (1979), 'Contribution from geriatric medicine within acute medical wards', *British Medical Journal*, 14 July, 90–94.

Burns, T. and Stalker, G.M. (1961), *The Management of Innovation*, Tavistock, London.

Butler, A., Oldman, C. and Grieve, J. (1983), *Sheltered Housing for the Elderly*, Allen and Unwin, London.

Butler, A., Oldman, C. and Wright, R. (1979), *Sheltered Housing for the Elderly: A Critical Review*, University of Leeds.

Bytheway, B. and James, L. (1978), *The Allocation of Sheltered Housing: A Study of Theory, Practice and Liaison*, Medical Sociology Research Centre, University of Swansea.

Cang, S. (1978), 'Full-time and part-time patients: An analysis of patient needs and their implications for domiciliary and institutional care', in Jacques, E. (ed.), *Health Services*, Heinemann Educational Books, London.

Carboni, D.K. (1982), *Geriatric Medicine in the United States and Great Britain*, Greenwood Press, Westport, Conn.

Carter, J. (1981), *Day Services for Adults*, Allen and Unwin, London.

Castle, B. (1980), *The Castle Diaries*, Weidenfeld and Nicholson, London.

Central Statistical Office (1984), *Social Trends*, 14, HMSO, London.

Challis, D.J. and Davies, B.P. (1986), *Case Management in Community Care*, Gower, Aldershot.

Challis, L. (1985), 'Controlling for care: Private and voluntary homes registration and inspection: A forgotten area of social work', *British Journal of Social Work*, 15:1, 43–57.

Child, J. (1972), 'Organisational structure, environment and performance: The role of strategic choice', *Sociology*, 6:1, 1–22.

Chisholm, I. and Fletcher, P. (1979), *The Park Club: A study of a club run by voluntary effort to help support confused elderly people and their families*, Buckinghamshire SSD, Aylesbury.

Cmnd 3703 (1968), *Local Authority and Allied Social Services* (Report of the Seebohm Committee), HMSO, London.

Cmnd 6951 (1977), *Housing Policy: A Consultative Document*, HMSO, London.

Cmnd 8173 (1981), *Growing Older*, HMSO, London.

Cmnd 8494 (1982), *The Government's Expenditure Plans*, 1982–83 to 1984–5, HMSO, London.

Congressional Budget Office (1981), *The Impact of PSROs on Health Care Costs: Update of Congressional Budget Office's 1979 Evaluation*, Government Printing Office, Washington, DC.

Cooper, B. and Bickel, H. (1984), 'Population screening and the early detection of dementing disorders in old age: A review', *Psychological Medicine*, 14, 81–95.

Cooper, M. (1980), 'Normanton: Interweaving social work and the community', in Hadley, R. and McGrath, M. (eds), *Going Local*, Bedford Square Press, London.

Crosbie, D. (1983), 'A role for anyone? A description of social work with the elderly in two area offices', *British Journal of Social Work*, 13, 123–48.

Dartington, T. (1978), *Volunteers and Psychiatric Aftercare*, Volunteer Centre, Berkhamsted.

Davies, B.P. (1981a), *A Policy Accident and the Regulatory Response*, Discussion Paper 165, Personal Social Services Research Unit, University of Kent, Canterbury.

Davies, B.P. (1981b), 'Strategic goals and piecemeal innovations', in Goldberg, E.M. and Hatch, S. (eds), *A New Look at the Personal Social Services*, Policy Studies Institute, London.

Davies, B.P. (1986), 'American lessons for British policy and research on long-term care of the elderly', *The Quarterly Journal of Social Affairs*, 2:3, 321–55.

Davies, B.P., Barton, A. and McMillan, I. (1972), *Variations in Children's Services Amongst British Urban Authorities*, Bell, London.

Davies, B.P., Barton, A., McMillan, I. and Williamson, V.K. (1971), *Variations in Services for the Aged*, Bell, London.

Davies, B.P. and Challis, D.J. (1986), *Matching Resources to Needs in Community Care*, Gower, Aldershot.

Davies, B.P. and Ferlie, E.B. (1982), 'Efficiency promoting innovation in social care: SSDs and the elderly', *Policy and Politics*, 10, 181–205.

Davies, B.P. and Ferlie, E.B. (1984), 'Patterns of efficiency improving innovations: Social care and the elderly', *Policy and Politics*, July, 281–95.

De Largy, J. (1957), 'Six weeks in: Six weeks out', *Lancet*, 23 February, 418–19.

Department of Health and Social Security (1970), *Circular 5/70: Organisation of Meals-on-Wheels*, HMSO, London.

Department of Health and Social Security (1971), *Circular 53/71: Help in the Home: Section 13 of the Health Services and Public Health Act*, HMSO, London.

Department of Health and Social Security (1976a), *Priorities for Health and Personal Social Services*, HMSO, London.

Department of Health and Social Security (1976b), *The NHS Planning System*, HMSO, London.

Department of Health and Social Security (1978), *A Happier Old Age*, HMSO, London.

Department of Health and Social Security (1983), *Care in the Community*, HC(83)6, LAC(83)5, HMSO, London.

Dickson, N. (1980), *Age Concern at Work*, Age Concern, London.

Donabedian, A. (1982), *The Criteria and Standards of Quality*, Health Administration Press, Ann Arbor, Michigan.

Donnison, D., Chapman, V., Meacher, M., Sears, A. and Urwin, K. (1975), *Social Policy and Administration Revisited*, Allen and Unwin, London.

Eaton Griffith, V. and Miller, C. (1980), 'Volunteer stroke scheme for dysphasic patients with stroke', *British Medical Journal*, 281, 1605–7.

Edwards, C., Sinclair, I. and Gorbach, P. (1980), 'Day centres for the elderly: Variations in type, provision and user response', *British Journal of Social Work*, 10, 419–30.

Equal Opportunities Commission (1982), *Caring for the Elderly and Handicapped: Community Care and Women's Lives*, EOC, Manchester.

Evans, J.G. (1981), 'Hospital services for the elderly', in Shegog, R.F.A. (ed.), *The Impending Crisis of Old Age*, Oxford University Press, Oxford.

Fennell, G. (1977), 'Social Interaction in Grouped Dwellings for the Elderly', BSA Social Policy Study Group Paper, unpublished.

Fennell, G., Emerson, A.R., Sidell, M. and Hague, A. (1981), *Day Centres for the Elderly in East Anglia*, University of East Anglia, Norwich.

Ferlie, E.B. (1982), *Sourcebook of Innovations in the Community Care of the Elderly*, Discussion Paper 261, Personal Social Services Research Unit, University of Kent, Canterbury.

Ferlie, E.B., Challis, D.J. and Davies, B.P. (1980), *Directory of Initiatives in Community Care for the Elderly*, Discussion Paper 148, Personal Social Services Research Unit, University of Kent, Canterbury.

Ferlie, E.B., Challis, D.J. and Davies, B.P. (1983), *A Guide to Efficiency-Improving Innovations in the Care of the Frail Elderly*, Discussion Paper 284, Personal Social Services Research Unit, University of Kent, Canterbury.

Ferlie, E.B., Challis, D.J. and Davies, B.P. (1984), 'Models of innovation in the social care of the elderly', *Local Government Studies*, November/December, 67–82.

Ferlie, E.B., Challis, D.J. and Davies, B.P. (1985), 'Innovation in the care of the elderly: the role of joint finance', in Butler, A. (ed.), *Ageing: Recent Advances and Creative Responses*, Croom Helm, London.

Ferlie, E.B., Challis, D.J. and Davies, B.P. (1988), *Efficiency-Improving Innovations in the Community Care of Frail Elderly People: Individual Schemes and their Characteristics*, Personal Social Services Research Unit, University of Kent, Canterbury.

Finch, J. (1984), 'Community care: Developing non-sexist alternatives', *Critical Social Policy*, 9, 6–18.

Finch, J. and Groves, D. (1983), *A Labour of Love*, Routledge and Kegan Paul, London.

Foster, E.M, Kay, D.W.K. and Bergmann, K. (1976), 'The characteristics of old people receiving and needing domiciliary services: The relevance of psychiatric diagnosis', *Age and Ageing*, 5, 245–55.

Fox, D. (1981), 'Housing and the elderly', in Hobman, D. (ed.), *The Impact of Ageing*, Croom Helm, London.

Frankfather, D.L., Smith, M.J. and Caro, F.G. (1981), *Family Life of the Elderly*, Heath, Lexington, Mass.

Gladstone, F.J. (1979), *Voluntary Action in a Changing World*, Bedford Square Press, London.

Glennerster, H., Korman, N. and Marslen-Wilson, F. (1983), 'Plans and practice: The participants' views', *Public Administration*, 61, 253–64.

Glennerster, H., Korman, N., Marslen-Wilson, F. and Meredith, B. (1982), *Social Planning: A Local Study*, London School of Economics and Political Science.

Goldberg, E.M. and Connelly, N. (1982), *The Effectiveness of Social Care for the Elderly*, Heinemann Educational Books, London.

Goldberg, E.M., Mortimer, A. and Williams, B.T. (1970), *Helping the Aged*, Allen and Unwin, London.

Goldberg, E.M. and Warburton, R.W. (1979), *Ends and Means in Social Work*, Allen and Unwin, London.

Grad, J. and Sainsbury, P. (1968), 'The effects patients have on their families in a community care and a control psychiatric service: A two year follow-up', *British Journal of Psychiatry*, 114, 265–8.

Grant, G. (1981a), *Monitoring Social Services Delivery in Rural Areas: Intake Cases in Two Contrasting Teams*, University College of North Wales, Bangor.

Grant, G. (1981b), *Monitoring Social Services Delivery in Rural Areas:*

Long-term Work in Two Contrasting Area Teams, University College of North Wales, Bangor.

Griffiths, R. (1988), *Community Care: Agenda for Action*, HMSO, London.

Gwynne, D. (1980), 'Home help service in Cumbria', in Social Services Research Group, *Research and Policy Making in the Home Help Service*, Report of a Conference.

Gwynne, D. and Fean, L. (1978), *The Home Help Service in Cumbria*, Cumbria SSD, Carlisle.

Hadley, R., Dale, P. and Sills, P. (1984), *Decentralising Social Services*, Bedford Square Press, London.

Hadley, R. and McGrath, M. (1984), *When Services are Local: The Normanton Experience*, National Institute for Social Work, London.

Hadley, R., Webb, A.L. and Farrell, C. (1975), *Across the Generations*, Allen and Unwin, London.

Hage, J. (1980), *Theories of Organization*, Wiley, New York.

Hage, J. and Dewar, R. (1973), 'Elite values versus organisational structure in predicting innovation', *Administrative Science Quarterly*, 18, 279–90.

Harbert, W. and Dexter, M. (1983), *The Home Help Service*, Tavistock, London.

Hasenfeld, Y. (1983), *Human Services Organizations*, Prentice Hall, Englewood Cliffs, New Jersey.

Hatch, S. (1980), *Outside the State*, Croom Helm, London.

Hatch, S. and Mocroft, I. (1979), 'The relative costs of service provided by voluntary and statutory organisations', *Public Administration*, 57:4, 393–405.

Health Advisory Service (1983), *The Rising Tide*, HMSO, London.

Hearnden, D. (1983), *Continuing Care Communities: A Viable Option in Britain?*, Centre for Policy in Ageing, London.

Hedley, R. and Norman, A. (1982), *Home Help: Key Issues in Service Provision*, Centre for Policy on Ageing, London.

Hemsi, L. (1981), *Jubilee Unit for the Psychiatry of Old Age*, Springfield Hospital, London.

Hemsi, L. (1982), 'Psychogeriatric care in the community', in Levy, R. and Post, F. (eds), *The Psychiatry of Late Life*, Blackwell, Oxford.

Heumann, L. and Boldy, D. (1982), *Housing for the Elderly*, Croom Helm, London.

Hey, A. (1980), 'Providing basic services at home', in Billis, D.,

Bromley, G., Hey, A. and Rowbottom, R. (eds), *Organising Social Service Departments*, Heinemann Educational Books, London.

Hildick-Smith, M. (1980), 'Geriatric day hospitals: Practice and planning', *Age and Ageing*, 9, 38–46.

Holme, A. and Maizels, J. (1978), *Social Workers and Volunteers*, Allen and Unwin, London.

Hood, C. and Dunsire, A. (1981), *Bureaumetrics*, Gower, Aldershot.

House of Commons Select Committee on the Social Services (1984), *Public Expenditure on the Social Services*, Session 1983–4, HCP395, 395-i and 395-ii, HMSO, London.

Howell, N., Boldy, D. and Smith, B. (1979), *Allocating the Home Help Service*, Bell, London.

Hunt, A. (1978), *The Elderly at Home*, HMSO, London.

Hurley, B. and Wolstenholme, L. (1980), 'The home help study: A summary of the findings and implications of the (Bradford) social services research project', *Clearing House for Local Authority Social Services Research*, 1, 35–70.

Hyman, M. (1981), *The Home Help Service: A Case History Study in the London Borough of Redbridge*, Redbridge SSD.

Isaacs, B. (1981), 'Is geriatrics a specialty?', in Arie, T. (ed.), *Health Care of the Elderly*, Croom Helm, London.

Isaacs, B., Livingstone, M. and Neville, Y. (1972), *Survival of the Unfittest*, Routledge and Kegan Paul, London.

Isaacs, B. and Neville, Y. (1976), *The Measurement of Need in Old People*, Scottish Health Services Studies No. 34, Scottish Home and Health Department, Edinburgh.

Johnson, M., di Gregorio, S. and Harrison, B. (1981), *Ageing — Needs and Nutrition: A Study of Voluntary and Statutory Collaboration in Community Care for Elderly People*, Policy Studies Institute, London.

Johnson, T. (1972), *Professions and Power*, Macmillan, London.

Kaim-Caudle, P. (1977), *The Sunderland Mobile Day Centre*, University of Durham.

Kay, D.W.K., Beamish, P. and Roth, M. (1964), 'Old age mental disorders in Newcastle-upon-Tyne: A study of prevalence', *British Journal of Psychiatry*, 110, 146–58.

Kay, D.W.K., Foster, E.M. and Garside, R.F. (1966), 'A four year follow-up study of a random sample of old people originally seen in their own homes: A physical, social and psychiatric enquiry', *Proceedings of the Fourth World Congress of Psychiatry*, Madrid, 1668–70.

Kay, J.A. (1985), 'Incomes of the elderly: The future of state provision', in R. Berthoud (ed.), *Challenges to Social Policy*, Gower, Aldershot.

Knapp, M. (1984), *The Economics of Social Care*, Macmillan, London.

Knapp, M. and Cambridge, P. (eds)(1988), *Demonstrating Successful Care in the Community*, Personal Social Services Research Unit, University of Kent, Canterbury.

Knapp, M. and Missiakoulis, S. (1982), 'Intersectoral cost comparisons: Day care for the elderly', *Journal of Social Policy*, 11:3, 335–55.

Kramer, R. (1981), *Voluntary Agencies in the Welfare State*, University of California Press, Berkeley.

Laing, W. (1985), *Private Health Care*, 1985, Office of Health Economics, London.

Levin, E., Sinclair, I. and Gorbach, P. (1982), *The Supporters of Confused Elderly Persons at Home*, National Institute for Social Work, London.

Lewis, J. (1976), 'Local Authority Health and Social Services in Four London Boroughs', Unpublished Ph.D. Thesis, University of London.

Lipman, A. (1967), 'Old people's homes: Siting and neighbourhood integration', *Sociological Review*, 15, 323–37.

Lipsky, M. (1980), *Street Level Bureaucracies*, Russell Sage, New York.

McAlpine, C.J. (1983), 'The geriatrician and the general practitioner', in F.I. Caird and J.G. Evans (eds), *Advanced Geriatric Medicine*, Pitman, London.

McArdle, C., Wylie, J.C. and Alexander, W.D. (1975), 'Geriatric patients in an acute medical ward', *British Medical Journal*, 5996, Vol. 4, 568–9.

Macdonald, R., Qureshi, H. and Walker, A. (1984), 'Sheffield shows the way', *Community Care*, 18 October, 28–30.

Means, R. (1981), *Community Care and Meals on Wheels: A Study in the Politics of Service Development at the National and Local Level*, Working Paper 21, School of Advanced Urban Studies, University of Bristol.

Mendel, J. (1979), 'Report to Family and Community Services on MIND's Woodhouse Project', Unpublished paper, Sheffield.

Ministry of Health (1957), *Circular 14/57: Local Authority Services for the Chronic Sick and Infirm*, HMSO, London.

Ministry of Housing and Local Government and Ministry of Health

(1961), *MHLG Circular 10/61*, MoH Circular 12/61: Services for Old People, HMSO, London.

Ministry of Housing and Local Government (1969), *Circular 82/69: Housing Standards and Costs — Accommodation Specially Designed for Old People*, HMSO, London.

Neill, J. (1981), 'Some Variations in Policy and Procedure Relating to Part III Admissions in the London Area', Unpublished paper, National Institute of Social Work, London.

Nissel, M. and Bonnerjea, L. (1982), *Family Care of the Handicapped Elderly: Who Pays?*, Policy Studies Institute, London.

Norman, A. (1982), *Mental Illness in Old Age: Meeting the Challenge*, Centre for Policy on Ageing, London.

Page, D. and Muir, T. (1971), *New Housing for the Elderly*, Bedford Square Press, London.

Parsloe, P. and Stevenson, O. (1978), *Social Services Teams: The Practitioners' View*, HMSO, London.

Pathy, J. (1982), 'Operational policies', in Coakley, D. (ed.), *Establishing a Geriatric Service*, Croom Helm, London.

Pettigrew, A.M. (1985), *The Awakening Giant*, Blackwell, Oxford.

Plank, D. (1977), *Caring for the Elderly*, Greater London Council, London.

Plank, M. (1982), *Teams for Mentally Handicapped People*, London, Campaign for Mentally Handicapped People, London.

Post, F. (1962), *The Significance of Affective Symptoms in Old Age*, Maudsley Monograph 10, Oxford University Press, Oxford.

Ratna, L. (1982), 'Crisis intervention in psychogeriatrics: A two year follow-up study', *British Journal of Psychiatry*, 141, 296–301.

Reid, W.J. and Shyne, A.W. (1969), *Brief and Extended Casework*, New York, Columbia University Press.

Renshaw, J., Hampson, R., Thomason, C., Darton, R., Judge, K. and Knapp, M. (1988), *Care in the Community: The First Steps*, Gower, Aldershot.

Rosow, I. (1967), *Social Integration of the Aged*, Free Press, New York.

Roth, M. and Kay, D.W.K. (1965), 'Affective disorders arising in the senium. Part 2: physical disability as an aetiological factor', *Journal of Mental Science*, 102, 141–50.

Rowlings, C. (1981), *Social Work with Elderly People*, Allen and Unwin, London.

Sanford, J. (1975), 'Tolerance of debility in elderly dependents at home: Its significance for hospital practice', *British Medical Journal*, 3, 471–3.

Schorr, A.L. (1970), 'The tasks for volunteerism in the new decade', *Child Welfare*, 49, 425–34.

Shenfield, B. and Allen, I. (1972), *The Organisation of Voluntary Service*, Broadsheet 533, Political and Economic Planning, London.

Sinclair, I., Levin, E., Neill, J., Gorbach, P. and Williams, J. (1986), 'Residential care: Applications and admissions', in Judge, K. and Sinclair, I. (eds), *Residential Care for Elderly People*, HMSO, London.

Social Services Inspectorate (1987), *From Home Help to Home Care: An Analysis of Policy, Resourcing and Service Management*, HMSO, London.

Stocking, B. (1985), *Initiative and Inertia*, Nuffield Provincial Hospitals Trust, London.

Stockport Housing Department (1980), *Special Housing Needs: Present and Future Policies*, Stockport County Council.

Thompson, M.K. (1981), 'Primary Care', in Shegog, R.F.A. (ed.), *The Impending Crisis of Old Age*, Oxford University Press, Oxford.

Thornton, P. and Moore, J. (1980), *The Placement of Elderly People in Private Households: An Analysis of Current Provision*, University of Leeds.

Tinker, A. (1980), *Housing the Elderly Near Relatives: Moving and Other Options*, Housing Development Directorate 1/80, Department of the Environment, London.

Tinker, A. (1984), *Staying at Home*, Department of the Environment, HMSO, London.

Townsend, P. (1962), *The Last Refuge*, Routledge and Kegan Paul, London.

Tunney, J. (1981), 'Hammersmith's initiatives 2: The housing management approach', *Housing Review*, 6, 93–5.

Vickery, A. (1981), *Consultation on 64 Cases of Elderly People Living Alone Referred for Social Work Help*, National Institute of Social Work, London.

Wagner, G. (1988), *Residential Care: The Research Reviewed*, HMSO, London.

Walker, G. (1975), 'Social networks in rural space: A comparison of two Southern Ontario localities', *East Lakes Geographer*, 10, 68–72.

Warwickshire SSD (1975), *Development of Sheltered Housing*, Warwickshire County Council, Warwick.

Warwickshire SSD (1980), *Your Own Front Door*, Warwickshire County Council, Warwick.

Webb, A.L. (1978), *Policy Innovation and the Balance of Social Care*, PSSRU/PSSC Conference on Developments in the Care of the Elderly, University of Kent, Canterbury.

Webb, A.L. (1985), 'Alternative futures for social policy and state welfare', in R. Berthoud (ed.), *Challenges to Social Policy*, Gower, Aldershot.

Weeks, D.R. (1973), 'Organisation theory: Some themes and distinctions', in G. Salaman and K. Thompson (eds), *People and Organizations*, Longman, London.

Wenger, C. (1982), 'Ageing in rural communities: Family contacts and community integration', *Ageing and Society*, 2:2, 211–30.

Wheeler, R. (1982), 'Staying put: A new development in policy?', *Ageing and Society*, 2:3, 299–329.

Willcocks, D., Peace, S. and Kellaher, L. (1982), *The Residential Life of Old People: A Study in 100 Local Authority Homes*, Polytechnic of North London, London.

Williams, A. and Anderson, R. (1975), *Efficiency in the Social Services*, Basil Blackwell, Oxford.

Williamson, J. (1981a), 'The preventive approach', in Kinnaird, J., Brotherston, J. and Williamson, J. (eds), *The Provision of Care for the Elderly*, Churchill Livingstone, Edinburgh.

Williamson, J. (1981b), 'Screening, surveillance and case finding', in Arie, T. (ed.), *Health Care of the Elderly*, Croom Helm, London.

Williamson, J., Stokoe, I., Gray, S., Fisher, M., Smith, A., Maghee, A. and Stephenson, E. (1964), 'Old people at home: Their unreported needs', *Lancet*, i, 1117–20.

Wolfenden, Lord (1978), *The Future of Voluntary Organisations*, Croom Helm, London.

Young, D. (1976), 'Provision of foster care services by voluntary agencies: Toward a theory of nonprofit organisations', *Urban Analysis*, 3, 29–59.

Young, D. and Finch, S. (1977), *Foster Care and Non Profit Agencies*, Lexington, New York.

Younghusband, E. (1959), *Report of the Working Party on Social Workers in the Local Authority Health and Welfare Services*, HMSO, London.

Younghusband, E. (1978), *Social Work in Britain*, 1950–1975, Allen and Unwin, London.

Author Index

207

Subject Index

210